POWER
ISO-BOW
ISOMETRIC
WORKOUTS XI

POWER ISO-BOW ISOMETRIC

WORKOUTS XI

The BEST Isometric programs that build muscle, burn fat, increase strength, all at home with the Iso-Bow

BECOME A ISOMETRIC POWERHOUSE

The Power Iso-Bow Isometric Workouts XI was written to help you get closer to your physical potential when it comes to real muscle sculpting strengthening exercises. The exercises and routines in this book are quite demanding, so consult your physician and have a physical exam taken prior to the start of this exercise program. Proceed with the suggested exercises and information at your own risk. The Publishers and author shall not be liable or responsible for any loss, injury, or damage allegedly arising from the information or suggestions in this book.

Power Iso-Bow Isometric Workouts XI
muscle-building Course

By

Birch Tree Publishing
Published by Birch Tree Publishing

Power Iso-Bow Isometric Workouts XI

© 2020 Copyright Birch Tree Publishing
Brought to you by the
Publishers of Birch Tree Publishing
ISBN-978-1-990089-05-3

Birch Tree Publishing

Dedication

For Popeye Spinach **POWER AND STRENGTH**, focus on **ISOMETRICS!**

Contents

GET "ISOMETRIC" STRONG

Introducing the worlds fastest strength, fat-loss producing system EVER!

Introduction by John Hughes

I have been involved with athletics all of my life, from college wrestling to World Championship Master's Wrestling in my 60s. Coupled with over 15 years of high school coaching, I have always strived for top physical performance in strength and flexibility for myself and the athletes I coached. I purchased my first Bullworker in the 1960s and was impressed with how quickly my body responded to Bullworker strength training. The portability of the product meant I never had to get rid of it due to space restraints and over the next 30 years, the ability to supplement any exercise routine with a quick Bullworker workout, always complimented my desired fitness goal.

In 1999, I became the North American distributor for Bullworker and began to work on design changes to make the product much more challenging, yet always maintaining the portability aspect of this time tested and proven fitness product. In recognizing the importance of cross-training principles for maximum fitness results, I designed additional products that kept with the Bullworker portability concept with each product able to be used either separately or combined for maximum fitness results in a complete cross-training program.

In 2010, I purchased most of the Global rights to Bullworker and have reintroduced Bullworker training principles that have been effective since 1962 and resulted in over 10 million units sold. Proven as the ultimate portable fitness products, Bullworker continues to deliver results to everyone, any age, wherever they exercise.

Today, I present the Iso-Bow Isometric Power Series. This book is about transforming your body, mind and spirit, which is what health, strength and physique enhancement is all about. I am really excited and positive to say that once you try the programs in this book, you will make some of the best gains you've ever made.
Join the men and women that are already using The Iso-Bow Isometric Power Series and programs with great success. **GET TRANSFORMED** today.

Keep pulling and pushing

Yours in Strength and Power

John Hughes

DEVELOP POWERFUL MUSCLES NOW

How Isometrics develops a powerful

Gain Popeye Strength levels with Isometrics

Chapter 1:

CHEST

CREATE A RIPPED CHEST

BUILD A RIPPED CHEST

01 BUILD A RIPPED CHEST

The chest muscles allow you to push or move the arm forward or across the body. These muscles are activated in any throwing or pushing motion. Aesthetically, building a powerful chest is a sign of power in men.

However, the chest muscles are not used daily, so most times they are under developed. So despite, the simplicity of how these muscles contract, they can be trained in a number of various angles of push and pull, each offer its own special muscle enhancing properties.

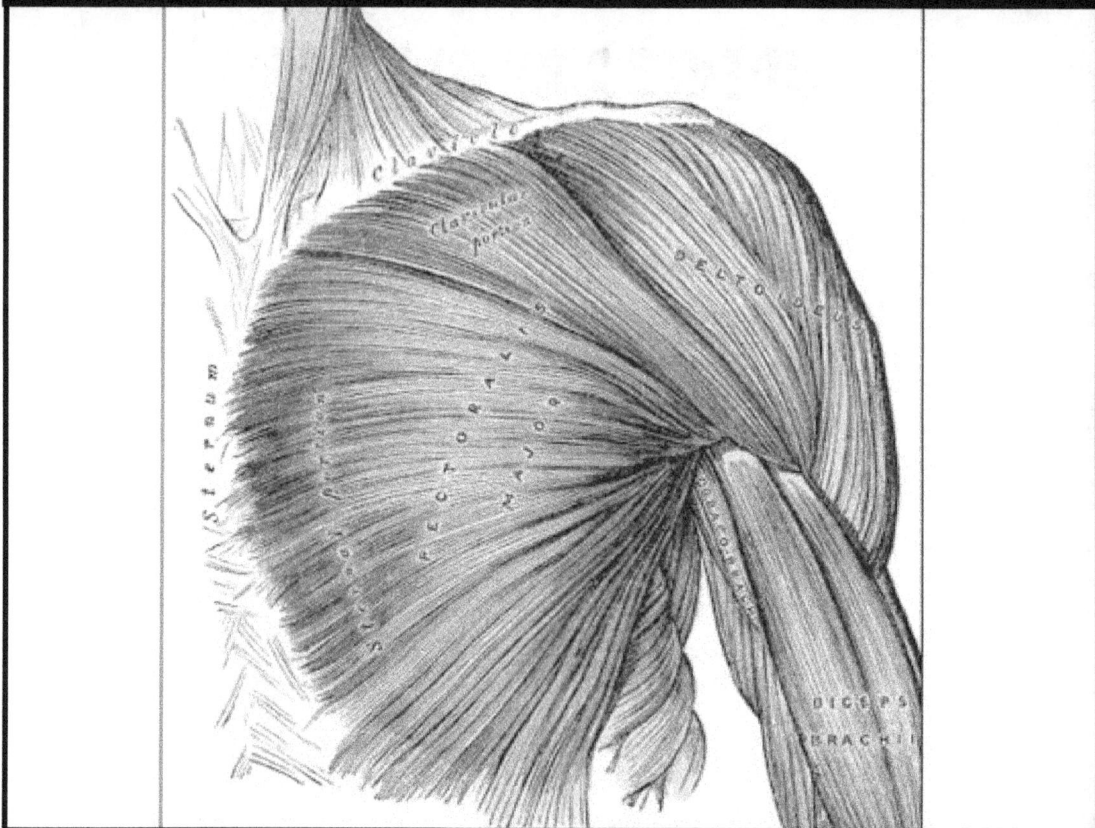

CHEST EXERCISES

01 BUILD A RIPPED CHEST

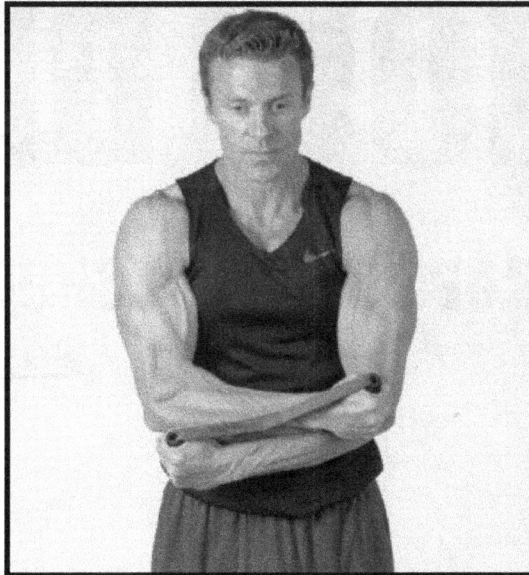

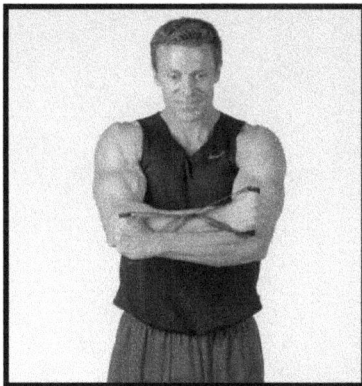

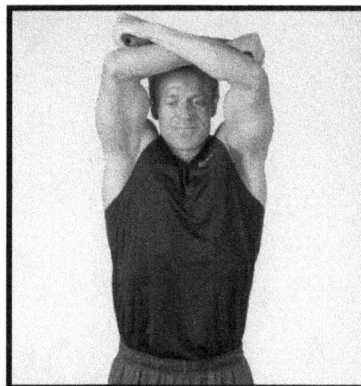

ISOMETRIC CHEST CONTRACTION

Cross arms as shown press the arms in opposite directions maintaining the tension. **(Isometric Contraction)** This exercise can be perform at various positions maintaining moderate tension.

Chapter 2:

SHOULDERS

DEVELOP POWERFUL SHOULDERS

DEVELOP POWERFUL SHOULDERS

02 DEVELOP POWERFUL SHOULDERS

The shoulder muscles are divided into three heads and are quite unique and move the arm in all directions. The front muscle raise the arm forward, the side muscles made up of a number of muscle bundles, and raises the arm out to the sides. The rear or posterior muscle, is designed to pull the arm backwards. Shoulder presses is a multi-muscle-use exercise, which is a compound exercise. This exercise recruits the front and side heads of the shoulders that tie in well with stimulating the upper and mid-back muscles as well giving the entire girdle complete development.

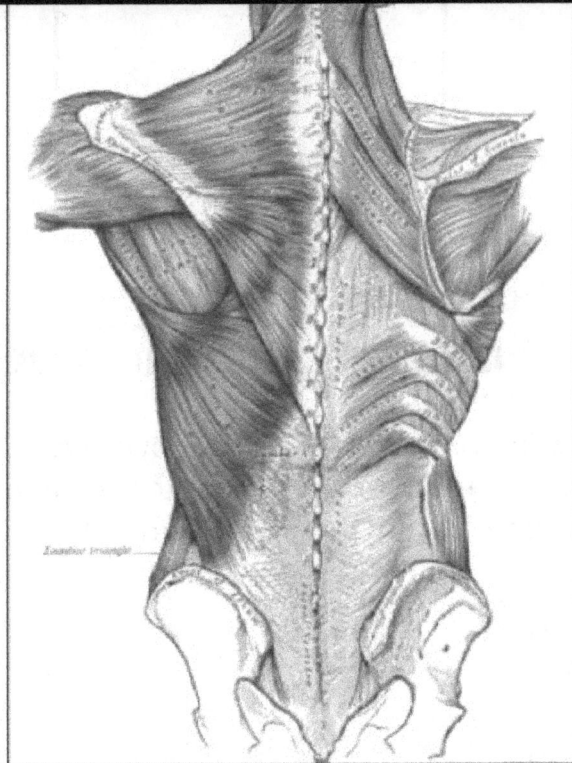

SHOULDER EXERCISES

02 DEVELOP POWERFUL SHOULDERS

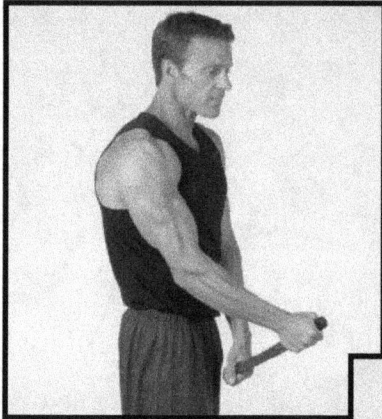

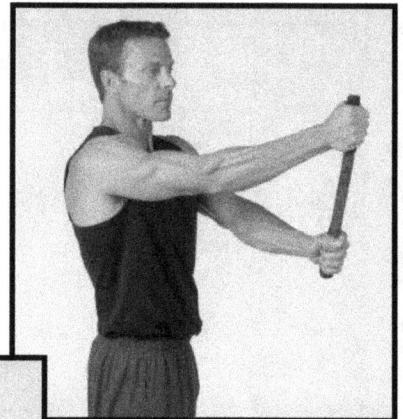

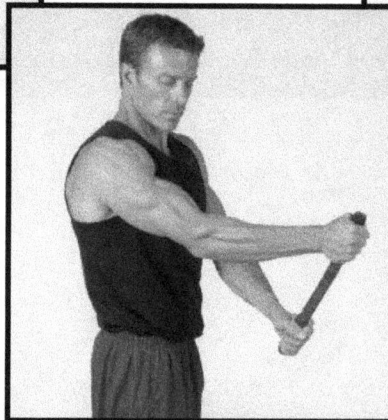

ISOMETRIC FORWARD CONTRACTION

Grasp the Iso-Bow in front of the body, as shown. We can do this movement at various angles for variety. Use moderate tension and keep breathing.
This works the front part of the shoulder muscles, along with the traps.

SHOULDER EXERCISES

02 DEVELOP POWERFUL SHOULDERS

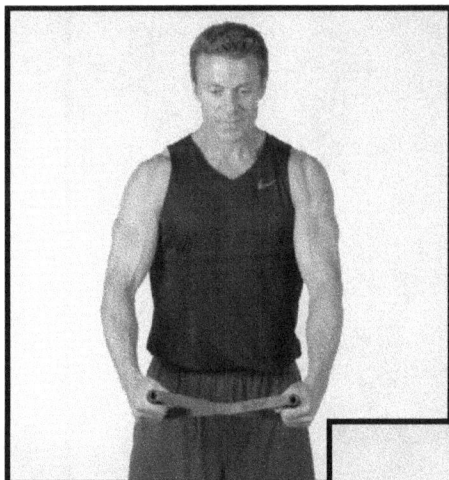

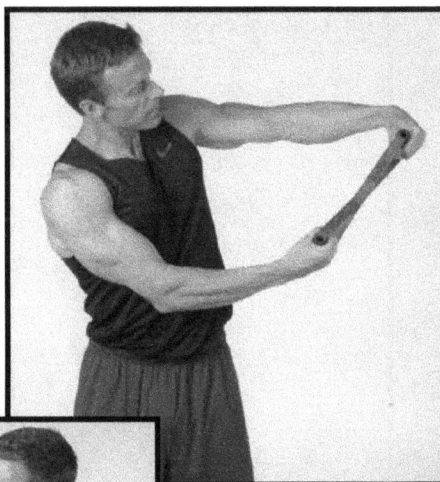

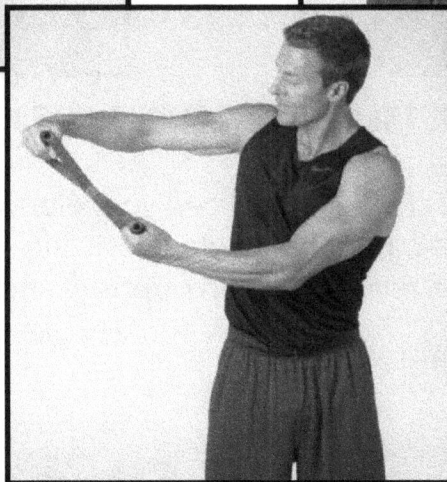

ISOMETRIC LATERAL RAISES

Hold the Iso-Bow at waist, keep your elbows slightly bent. We can do this movement at all three angles for variety. Use moderate tension and keep breathing.

SHOULDER EXERCISES

02 DEVELOP POWERFUL SHOULDERS

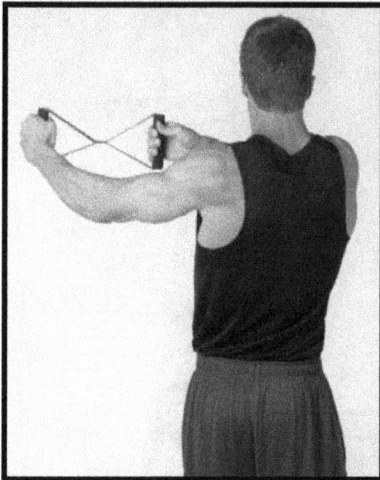

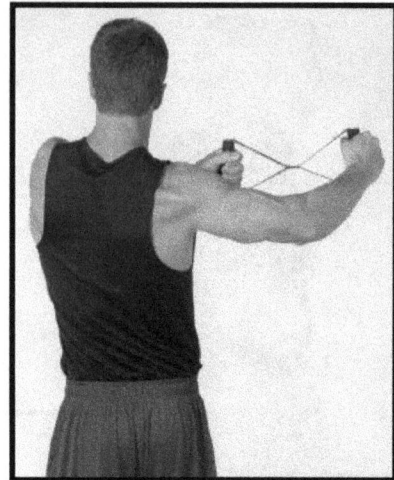

ACROSS THE BODY ISOMETRIC CONTRACTIONS

Place the Iso-Bow at chest height, keep your elbows slightly bent, pull Isometrically with the right hand while resisting with the other arm. Pause and reverse arms in opposite angle of pull.

Chapter 3:

UPPER BACK
DEVELOP A POWERFUL V-TAPER

DEVELOP A POWERFUL V-TAPER

03 DEVELOP A POWERFUL V-TAPER

The entire back is made up of many muscles overlapping each other. However, most trainees find the back quite difficult to fully develop. The reason? As the saying goes out of sight, out of mind. We cannot directly see the back muscles, plus we cannot see it flex like we would see the biceps.

We make training the entire back musculature much easier making developing the back obviously simple once you know what you are doing, you can bring these muscles up to speed. We are looking at the large Latissimus that covers the majority of the back. The trapezius is broken up into two sections.

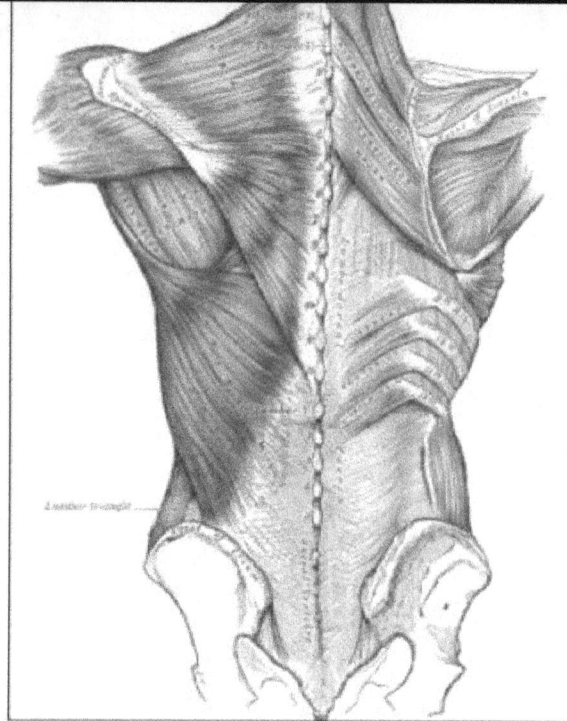

UPPER BACK EXERCISES

03 DEVELOP A POWERFUL V-TAPER

DO NOT NEGLECT THE MID AND LOWER TRAPS

The upper traps and mid-back muscles. Plus, we have the teres major, which is strongly stimulated with unilateral work, which makes isometrics the ideal movement. The infraspinatus muscle is like a half circle on each side of the upper back and is a very important rotator cuff muscle.

This muscle stabilizes the shoulder and prevents dislocations. Even though this muscle is at the back, most traditional exercises do not fully target these muscles. However, with our program there are exercises that target this area for full development.

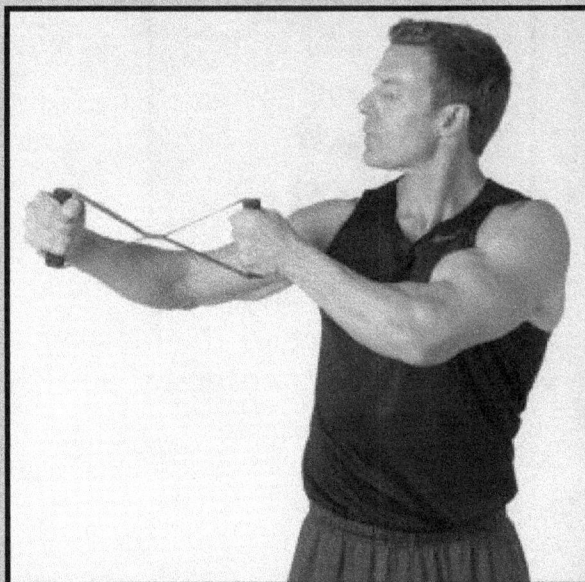

UPPER BACK EXERCISES

03 DEVELOP A POWERFUL V-TAPER

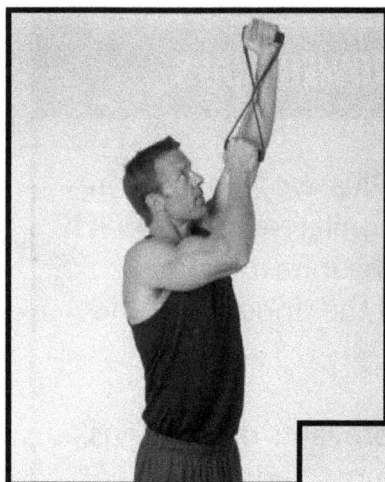

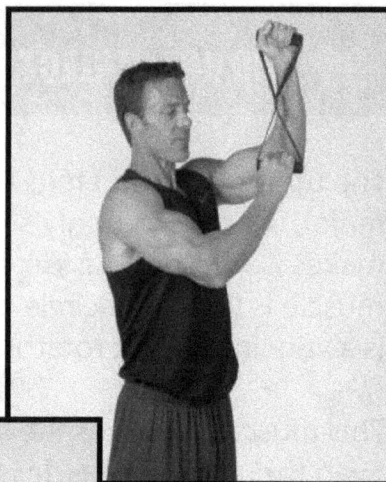

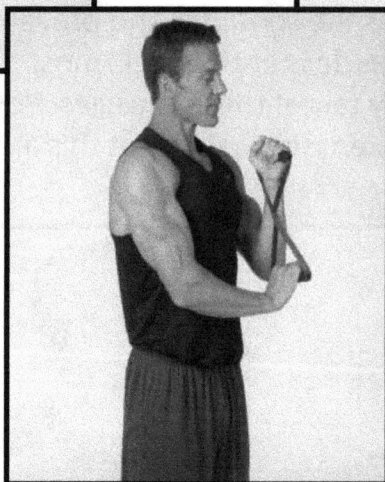

ISOMETRIC PULLDOWNS

Grasp the Iso-Bow as shown in the picture. This movement can be done at various angles for variety. Use moderate tension and keep breathing

UPPER BACK EXERCISES

03 DEVELOP A POWERFUL V-TAPER

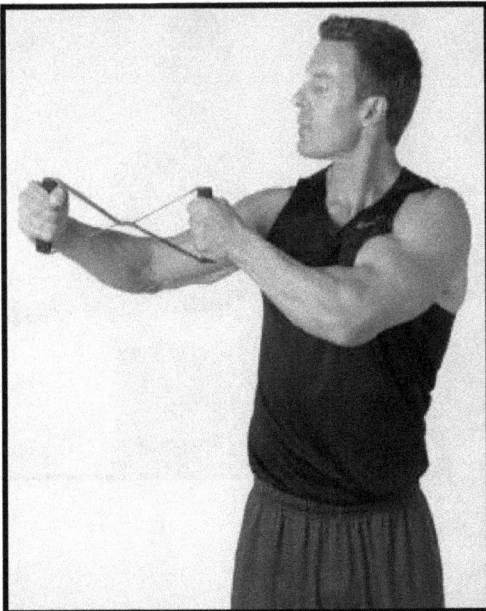

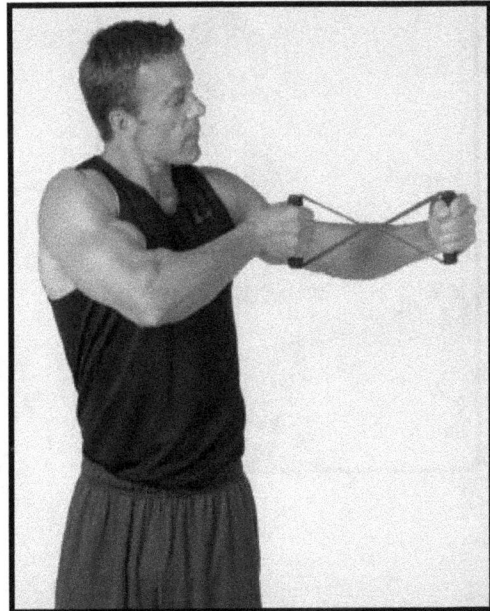

ISOMETRIC ROW

Bring your arm across the body pre-stretching the mid-back, grasp the Iso-Bow as shown. Pull in an isometric manner and hold. Switch arms and continue. Use moderate tension and keep breathing

UPPER BACK EXERCISES

03 DEVELOP A POWERFUL V-TAPER

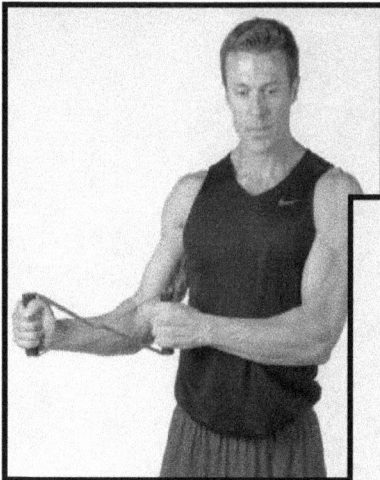

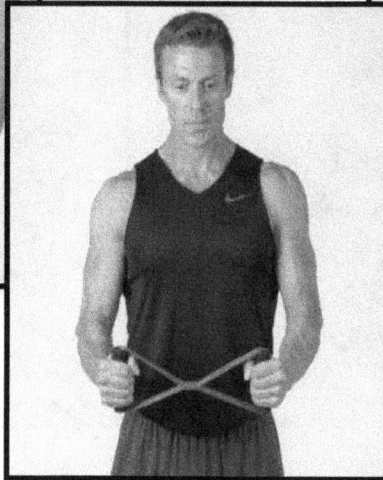

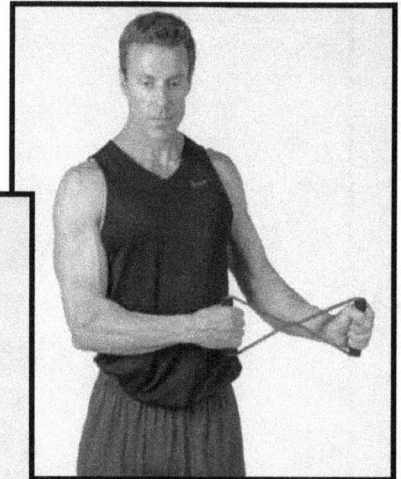

ADD ISOMETRIC POWER TO THE ROTATOR CUFF MUSCLES

Hold the Iso-Bow as shown. Pull with the left resisting isometrically with the right. This exercise can be done at various angles for variety. Use moderate tension and keep breathing

Chapter 4:

BICEPS
DEVELOP POWERFUL BICEPS

DEVELOP POWERFUL BICEPS

04 DEVELOP POWERFUL BICEPS

The biceps muscle has two heads. A short head, which is on the inside of the arm, and a long head, which is on the outside. This is the part that people see first. The main roll of the biceps is to flex the forearm by bringing the hand towards the shoulder. In order to build powerful complete biceps, you need to learn that the biceps do not work by itself.

The brachialis, which is under the bicep when developed, gives the bicep a larger and fuller appearance. Performing curls place undesirable tension on the tendon near the elbow. In other words, the biceps is placed in a very vulnerable position. Always start all bicep exercises with a slight bend at the start and finish. Always maintain tension on the biceps and not the joint.

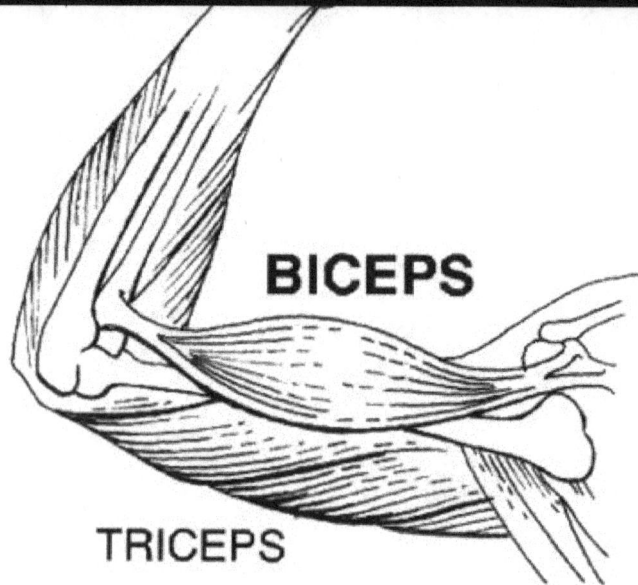

BICEPS

TRICEPS

BICEP EXERCISES

04 DEVELOP POWERFUL BICEPS

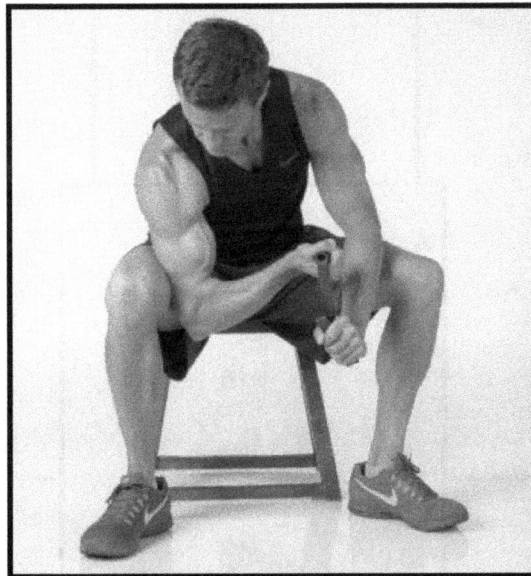

ISOMETRIC CONCENTRATION CURLS

As pictured, pull the right arm towards the face while resisting with the left hand Isometrically. Switch arms by pushing the left arm down and resisting with the right.

BICEP EXERCISES

04 DEVELOP POWERFUL BICEPS

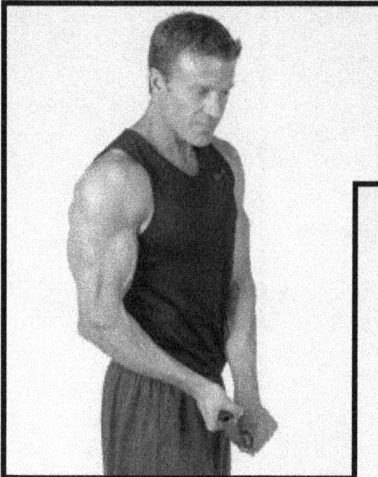

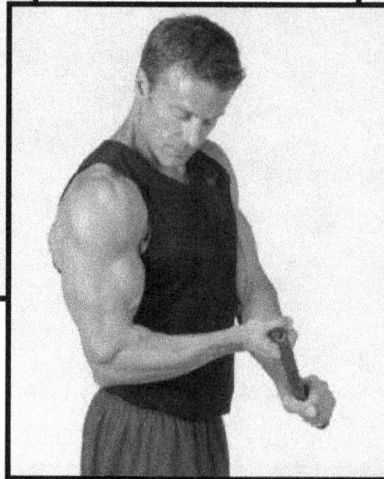

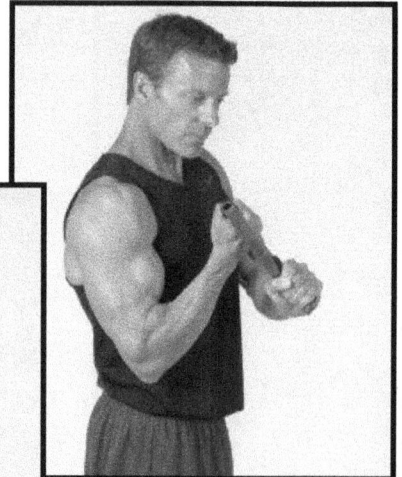

ISOMETRIC CURLS

Pull the right arm upward while resisting with the left hand Isometrically. Reverse arms and continue by pushing the left arm downwards, resisting with the right.

This movement can be done at various angles for variety. Use a moderate tension and keep breathing.

Chapter 5:

TRICEPS
DEVELOP POWERFUL TRICEPS

DEVELOP POWERFUL TRICEPS

05 DEVELOP POWERFUL TRICEPS

DEVELOP POWERFUL TRICEPS

The triceps has three heads: The lateral head, middle head and the long head. The role of the triceps is to straighten the arm. The triceps work in opposition to the biceps and brachialis muscles. The triceps has three heads this makes it much larger in mass than the biceps and the brachialis.

Unfortunately, most pay attention to the biceps, leaving the triceps underdeveloped. The lateral head, which is on the outside is what people see first. The triceps are easy to develop and we have made it easy for the trainee to achieve this.

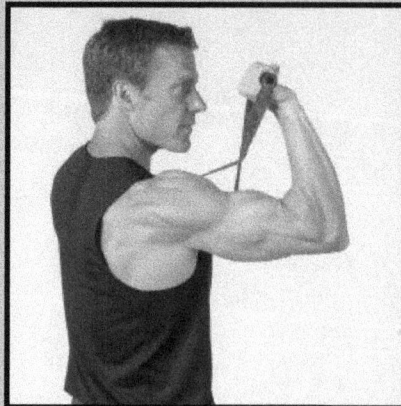

TRICEP EXERCISES

05 DEVELOP POWERFUL TRICEPS

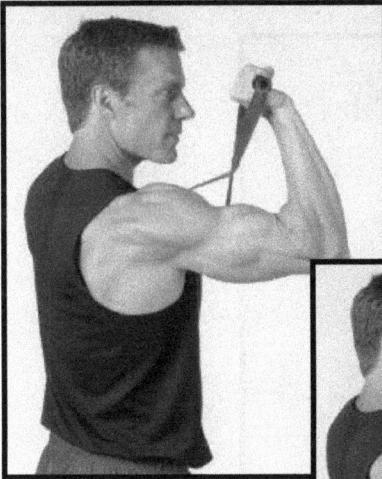

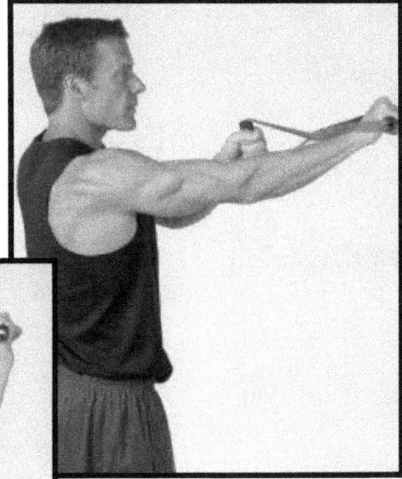

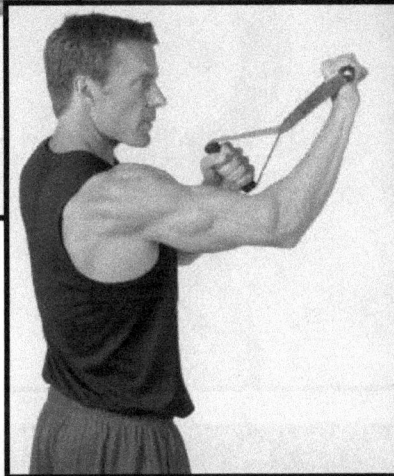

ISOMETRIC FORWARD EXTENSIONS

As shown above, push the right arm forward while resisting with the left hand **ISOMETRICALLY. Switch arms and repeat.**

TRICEP EXERCISES

05 DEVELOP POWERFUL TRICEPS

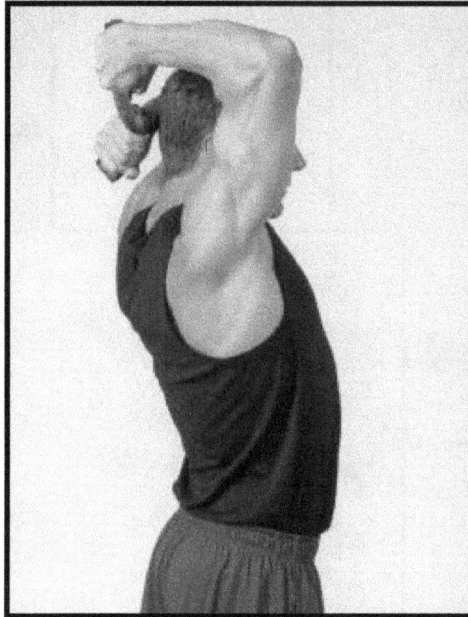

ISOMETRIC OVERHEAD TRICEP EXTENSIONS

Place arms overhead, press the right arm **ISOMETRICALLY** while resisting with the left arm. Use a light to moderate tension due to the tricep tendons being sensitive at this position.
SWITCH ARMS AND REPEAT

TRICEP EXERCISES

05 DEVELOP POWERFUL TRICEPS

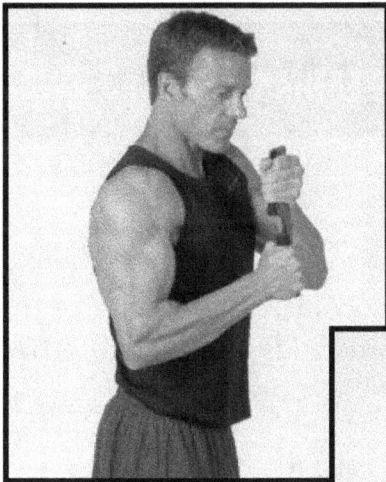

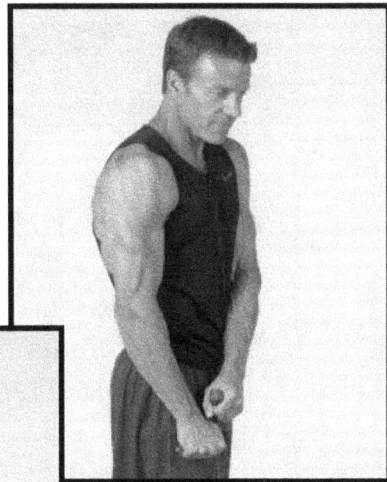

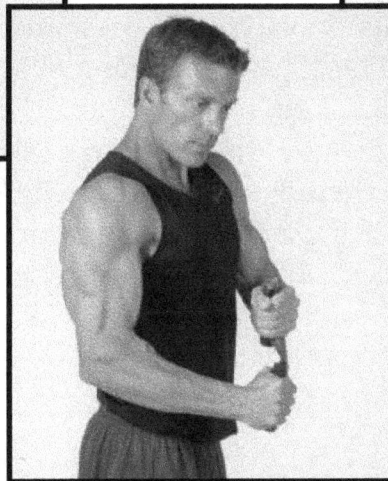

ISOMETRIC TRICEP PRESSDOWN

As pictured above, press the right hand downwards while resisting with the left arm. Change positions for variety. **RESIST ISOMETRICALLY**

DEVELOP RIPPED FOREARMS

06 DEVELOP RIPPED FOREARMS

DEVELOP RIPPED FOREARMS

DEVELOP RIPPED FOREARMS

Forearm muscles are involved in every daily activity, just like the calves and abdominals. We use these muscles all the time, when we drive, write, type, hold a bag and even open a door.

Many of the muscles of the forearm deal with Muscle-multi-use. When you are moving the elbow by lowering and raising the forearm. Moving the wrist up and down by, plus raising and lowering the hand. All Isometric exercises stress the forearms to contract which will increase your grip strength.

FOREARM EXERCISES

06 DEVELOP RIPPED FOREARMS

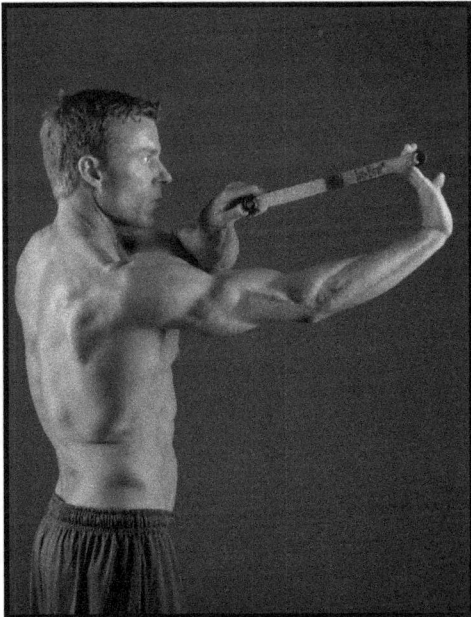

EXERCISE ONE

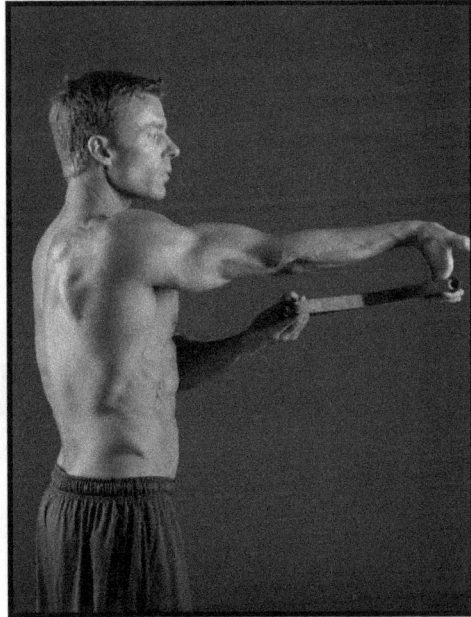

EXERCISE TWO

HAND/FOREARM EXERCISE

EXERCISE ONE: As pictured press the right hand forward. **RESIST ISOMETRICALLY.**

EXERCISE TWO: Same as exercise one but, the hand is placed downwards.

Chapter 7:

THIGHS
DEVELOP POWERFUL THIGHS

DEVELOP POWERFUL TIRELESS THIGHS

07 DEVELOP POWERFUL TIRELESS THIGHS

DEVELOP POWERFUL THIGHS

The thigh muscles are basically made up of four main muscles: the vastus lateral muscle, this is located on the outside of the thighs. The vastus medial muscle, this is located on the inside of the thigh muscles towards the knee.

Better known as the tear drop because of its shape. The recus-femoris, which is located in the center of the muscles, and the vastus intermedius, this muscle is mostly covered by all the other muscles of the thighs. Isometric contractions will develop tireless thighs with a power pack punch.

LEG EXERCISES

07 DEVELOP POWERFUL TIRELESS THIGHS

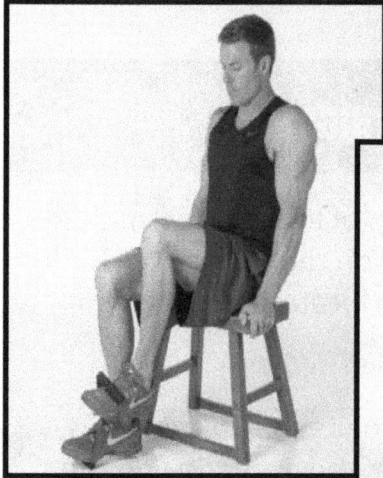

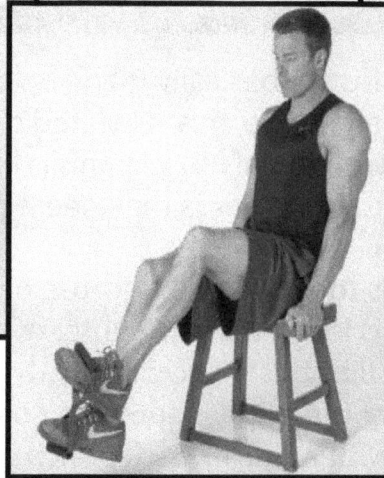

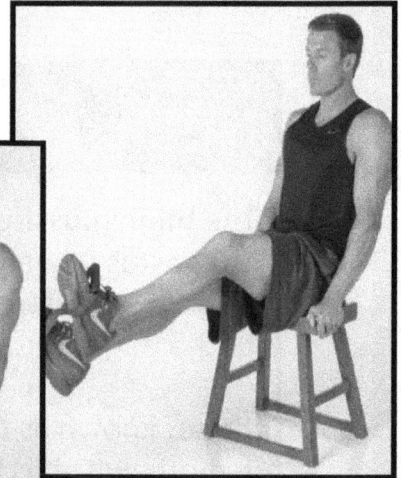

ISOMETRIC LEG EXTENSIONS

While seated on a chair, box or stool, place the legs as shown in the pictures. Maintain a Isometric static position for desired seconds, then switch legs. **RESIST ISOMETRICALLY**

LEG EXERCISES

07 DEVELOP POWERFUL TIRELESS THIGHS

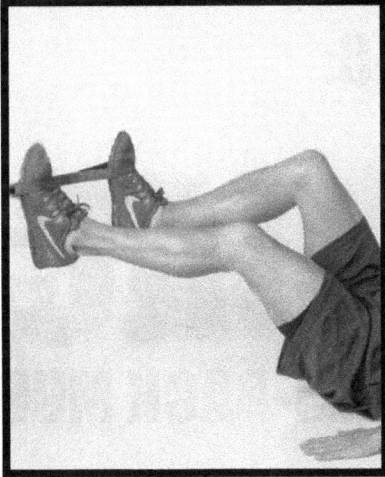

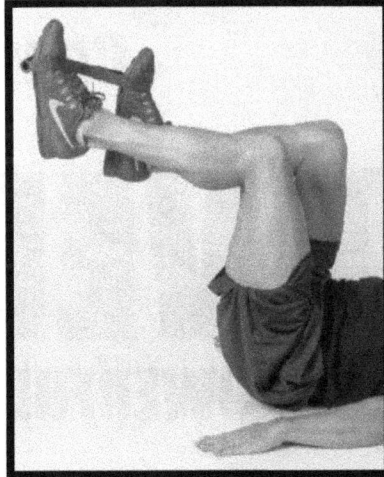

ISOMETRIC LEG PRESS

As shown, pull the right leg towards the chest, powerfully resisting with the left leg in a Isometric manner. Switch legs and continue.

Chapter 8:

LOWER-BACK
DEVELOP POWERFUL LOWER-BACK MUSCLES

DEVELOP POWERFUL LOWER BACK MUSCLES

08 DEVELOP POWERFUL LOWER-BACK MUSCLES

POWERFUL LOWER BACK MUSCLES

Develop Powerful Lower back muscles

The lower back muscles support the lower part of the spine. When these muscles are well developed it builds a brace protecting the spine.

Apart from that the lower back muscles are responsible for bringing the body upright from a leaning forward position. Not only will the lower back be involved, but the glutes and hamstrings come into play.

LOWER BACK EXERCISES

08 DEVELOP POWERFUL LOWER BACK

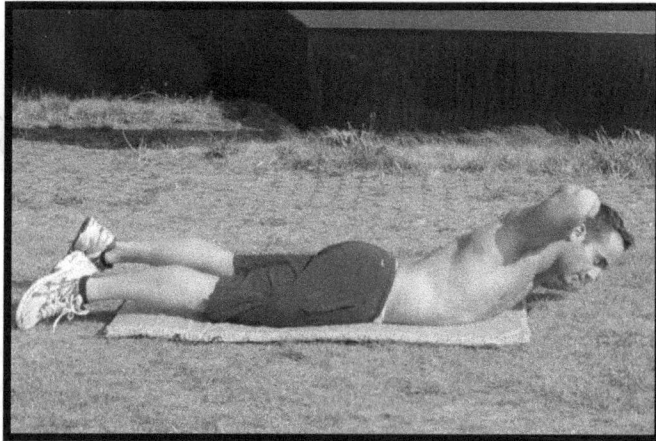

ISOMETRIC LOWER BACK EXTENSION

As shown above, lay flat on the floor and perform this movement by raising the upper body upwards and holding it Isometrically for the desired seconds.

Chapter 9:

CALVES
DEVELOP SHAPELY CALVES

DEVELOP SHAPELY CALVES

09 DEVELOP SHAPELY CALVES

DEVELOP SHAPELY CALVES

Develop shapely calves

The calves add a finished look to the lower leg with a diamond shape. This muscle has three heads (muscle parts) the soleus, this is under the large lateral head and gives the calves a fully developed look viewed from the side and back.

The lateral and medial heads are on the outside and in the middle of the muscle. The gastrocnemius make up the majority of the calf muscle. However, the longer the gastroc, the larger the potential for enhanced calf muscle development.

DEVELOP SHAPELY CALVES

09 DEVELOP SHAPELY CALVES

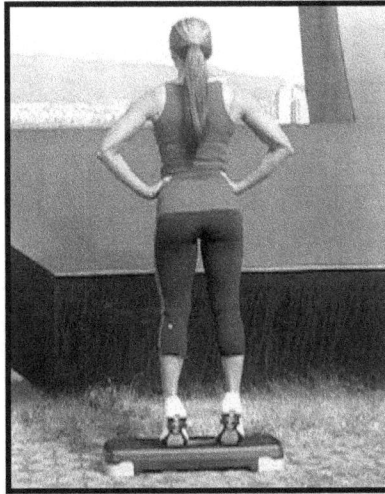

ISOMETRIC STANDING CALVE RAISES

Position yourself as shown but make sure the calves are contracted fully. Press straight up on the toes and hold the position Isometrically. This is a fantastic calve exercise.

Chapter 10:

ABDOMINALS
DEVELOP POWERFUL ABS

DEVELOP POWERFUL ABS

10 DEVELOP POWERFUL ABS

The abdominal muscles are very important and reveal that the trainee has a lean physique. Plus, the role of the abdominal muscles is to protect the spine. A lean chiseled set of abdominal muscles shows the opposite sex that the owner has a sign of virility.

Once these muscles are well developed this keeps the waist line and belly flat. There are various muscle structures that complete the overall look, the entire length of the abdominal wall, plus the internal and external obliques.

The lower sections of the abdominal muscles play the largest role in protecting the spine and storing belly fat. This is the easiest place for body-fat to accumulate. Which makes training with Isometric exercises ideal at stimulating those muscle fibers to the max.

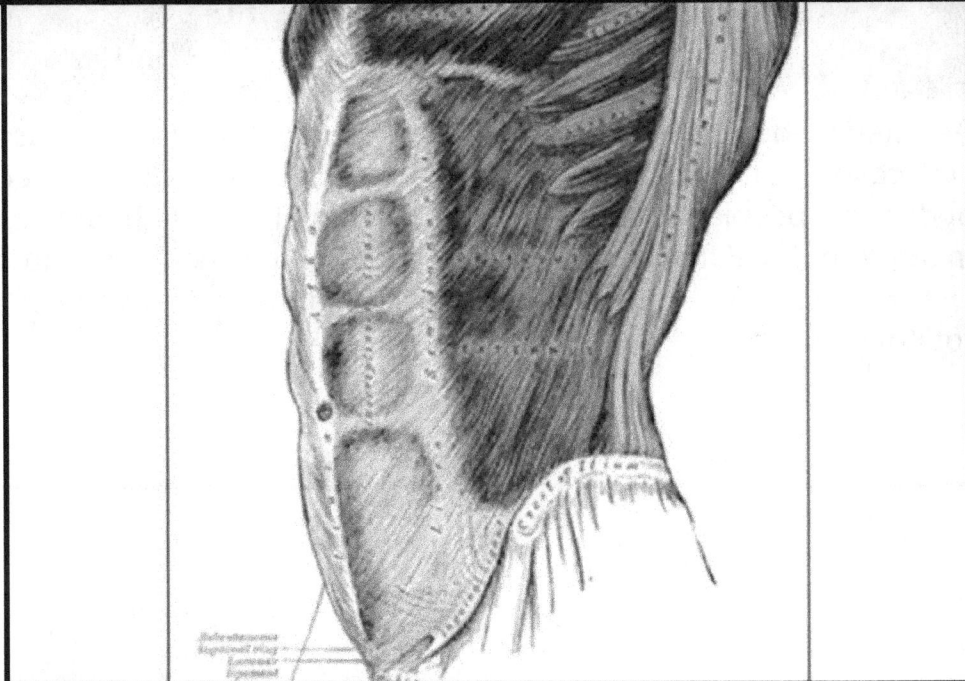

DEVELOP POWERFUL ABS

10 DEVELOP POWERFUL ABS

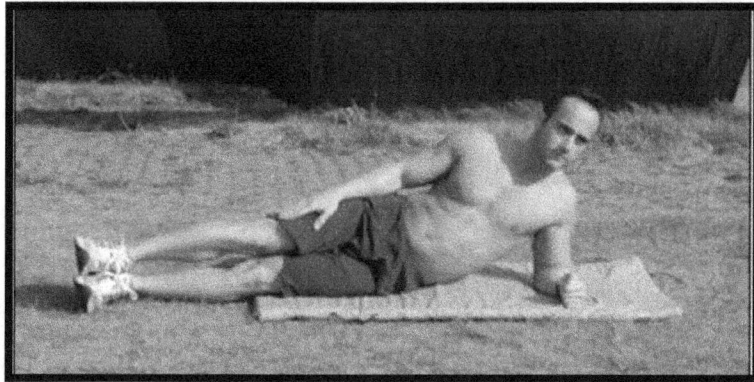

DEVELOP POWERFUL ABDOMINALS

As noted in the introduction the abdominal wall includes four muscles: Let's cover the entire length from the chest to pubis is called the rectus abdominis, people say abs for short. The abdominal wall should be worked in three angles of flexion. The lower sections of the abdominal muscles. The upper sections of the abdominal wall, and the obliques. Which are rotator muscles.

DEVELOP POWERFUL ABS

10 DEVELOP POWERFUL ABS

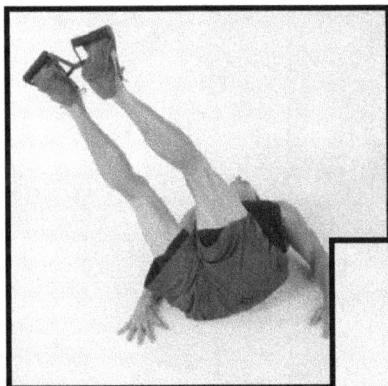
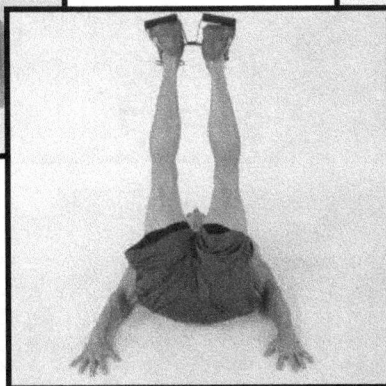
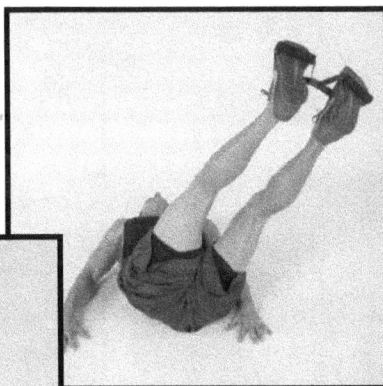

ISOMETRIC SIDE TO SIDE LATERAL ROTATIONS

Normally people say I want to get rid of my love handles. This Isometric abdominal exercise really isolates the entire ab dominal way as well as the oblique muscles.

These muscles support the spine by making the abdominal wall more rigid. Start off as shown, spread the Iso-Bow apart maintaining Isometric tension. Try the movement at various angles as shown.

DEVELOP POWERFUL ABS

10 DEVELOP POWERFUL ABS

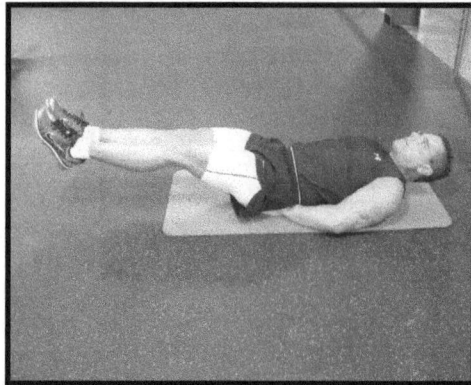

ISOMETRIC LEG HOLD

As shown above, place your hands under your butt and hold the position Isometrically for the desired seconds. This exercise stimulates the entire abdominal wall.

DEVELOP POWERFUL ABS

10 DEVELOP POWERFUL ABS

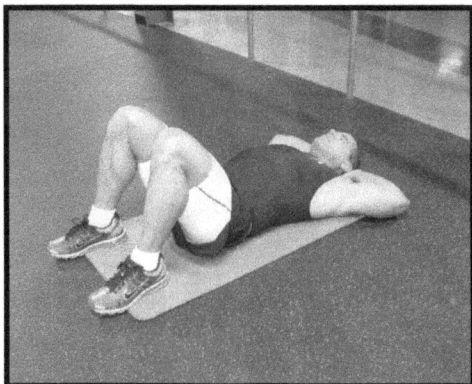

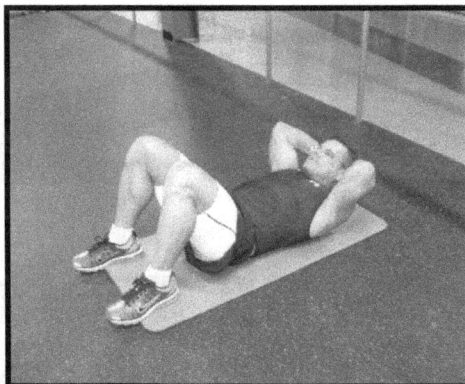

ISOMETRIC ABDOMINAL CRUNCHES

Lay on your back. Place the hands at your ear, tilt your head back, focus on the ceiling and go into the upward position as shown. **HOLD ISOMETRICALLY AND DO NOT PULL ON THE HEAD.**

Chapter 11:

POWER X PHASE ONE METHOD

PERFORM A 30 SECOND CONTRACTION AT 3 SETS, BEFORE MOVING ONTO THE NEXT EXERCISE ALL PHASES ARE TO BE PERFORMED FOR 2 WEEKS DO NOT SKIP PHASES

PHASE ONE

11 PHASE ONE

MONDAY, WEDNESDAY, FRIDAY

Perform a 30 second Isometric contraction, 3 sets each. Perform each exercise using 50% of force. Rest 5-10 seconds between sets.

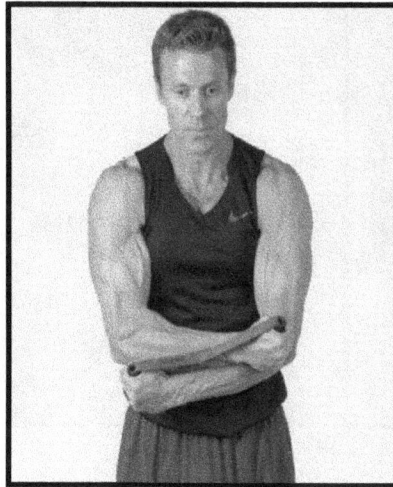

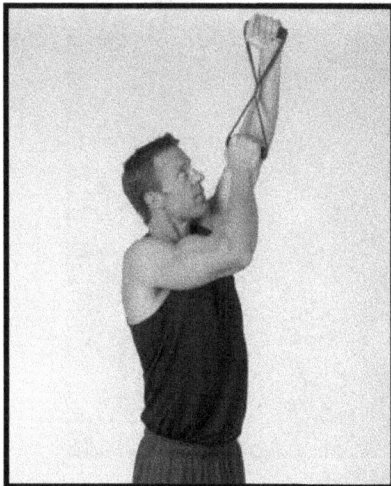

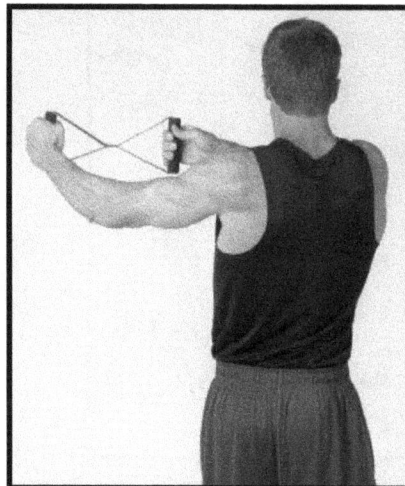

PHASE ONE

11 PHASE ONE

MONDAY, WEDNESDAY, FRIDAY
Routine continued.........

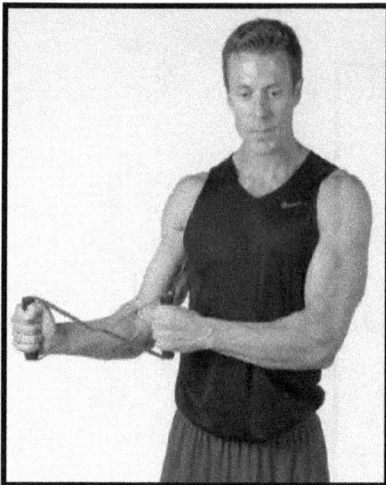

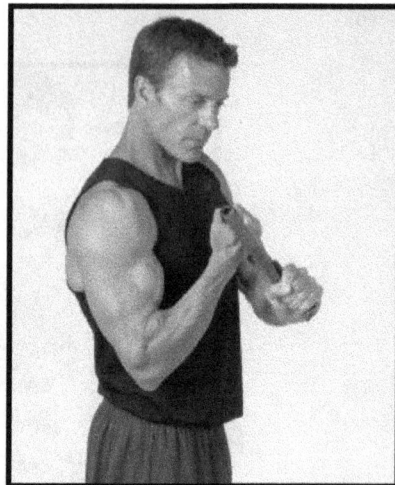

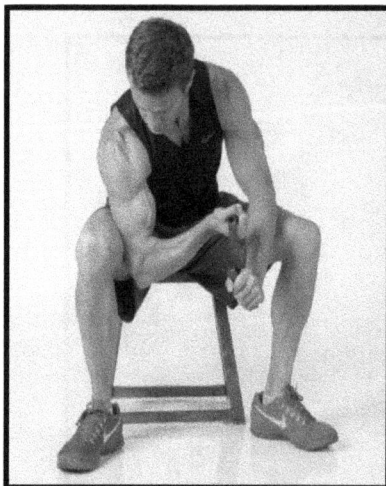

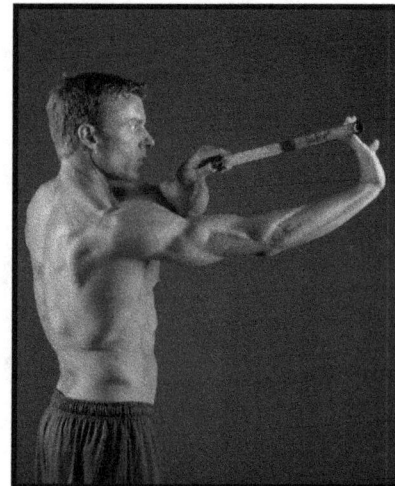

PHASE ONE

11 PHASE ONE

MONDAY, WEDNESDAY, FRIDAY
Routine continued...........

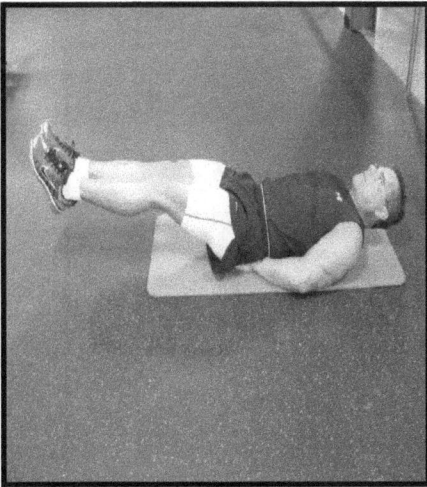

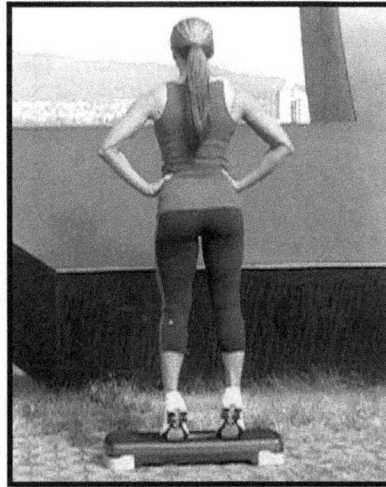

PHASE ONE MON, WED, FRI

PHASE ONE

11 PHASE ONE

TUESDAY, THURSDAY, SATURDAY

Perform a 30 second Isometric contraction, 3 sets each. Perform each exercise using 50% of force. Rest 5-10 seconds between sets.

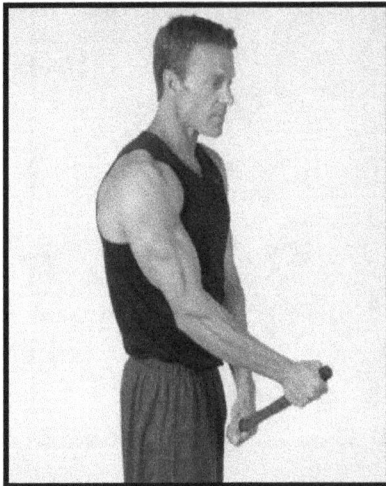

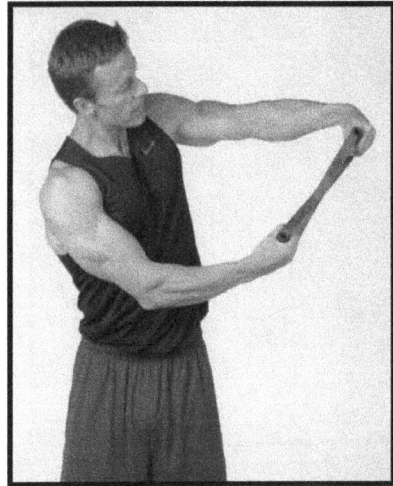

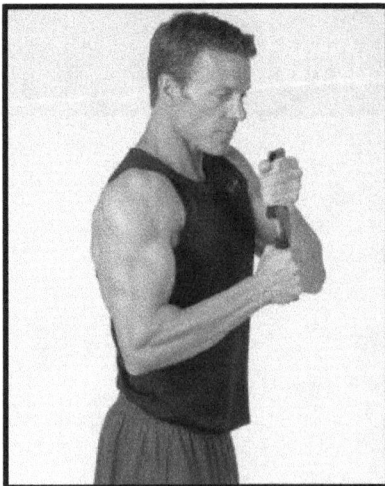

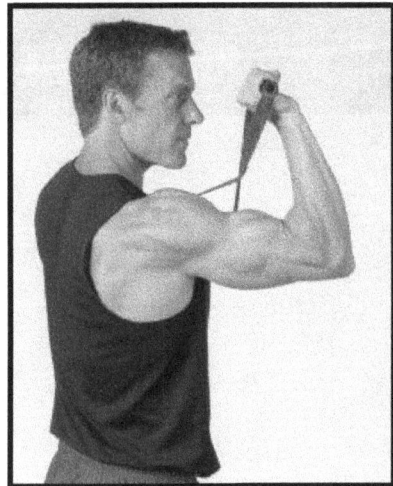

PHASE ONE

11 PHASE ONE

TUESDAY, THURSDAY, SATURDAY
Continued routine...........

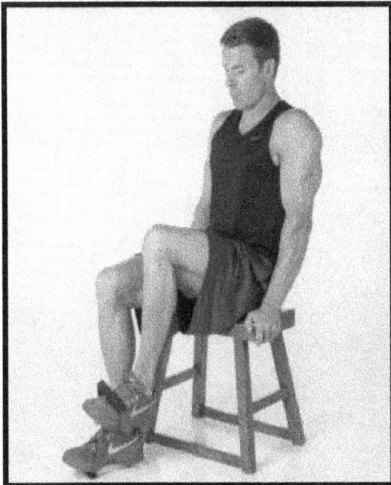

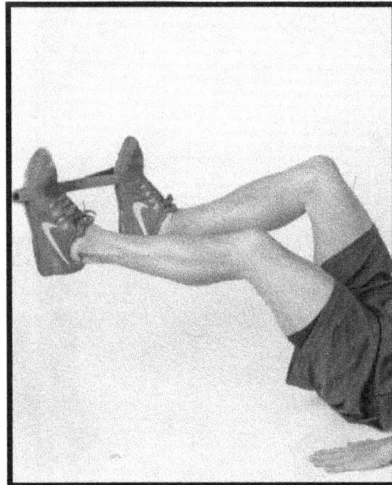

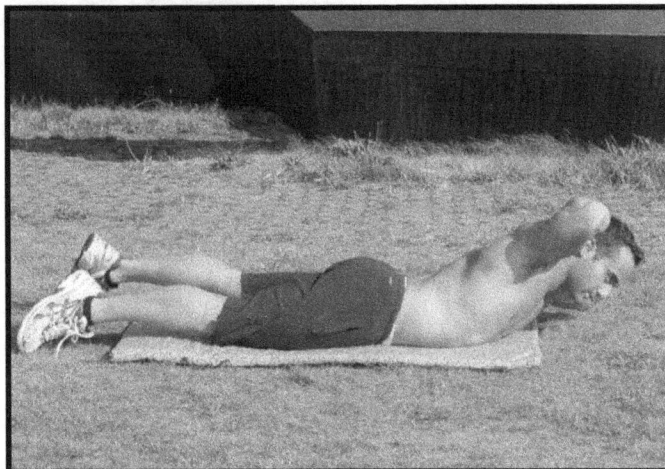

PHASE ONE

11 PHASE ONE

TUESDAY, THURSDAY, SATURDAY
Continued routine........

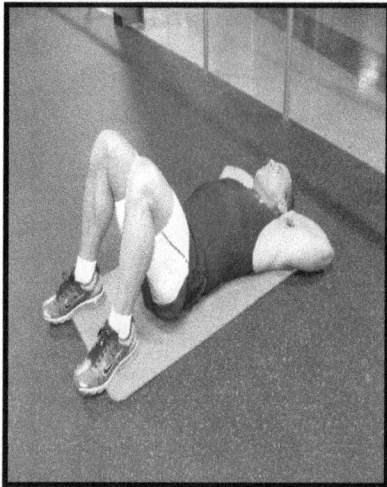

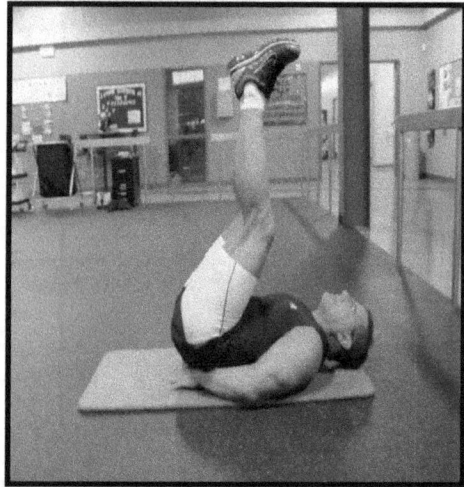

PHASE ONE TUES, THURS, SAT.

PHASE TWO

11 PHASE TWO

MONDAY, WEDNESDAY, FRIDAY

Perform a 20 second Isometric contraction, 3 sets each before moving to the next exercise. Perform each exercise using 50% of force.

PERFORM PROGRAM FOR 2 WEEKS

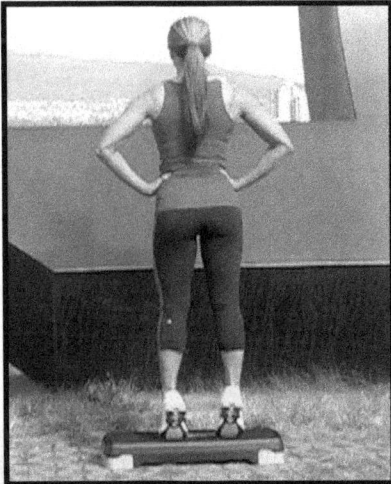

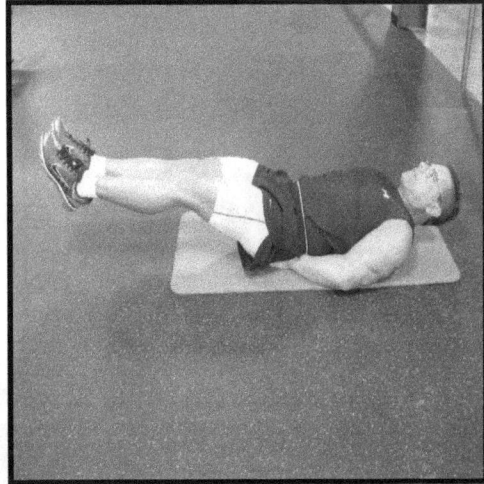

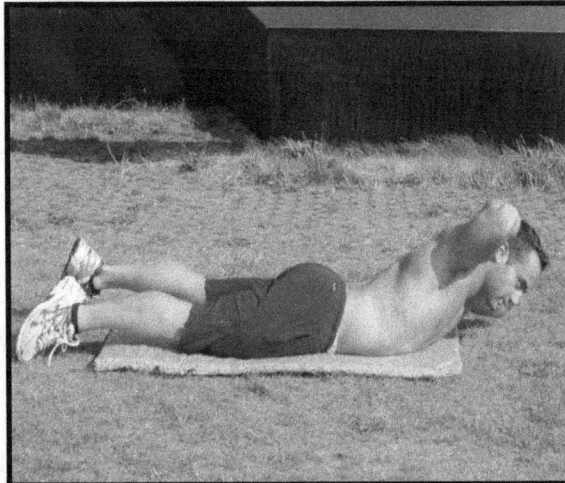

PHASE TWO

11 PHASE TWO

**MONDAY, WEDNESDAY, FRIDAY
ROUTINE CONTINUED........**

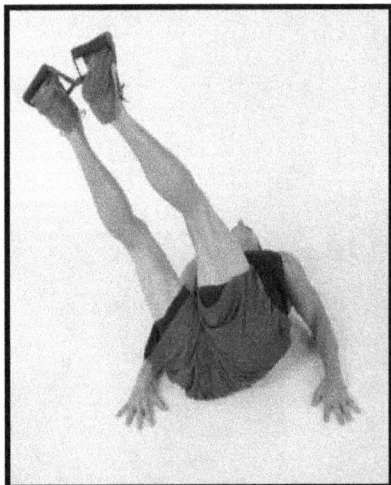

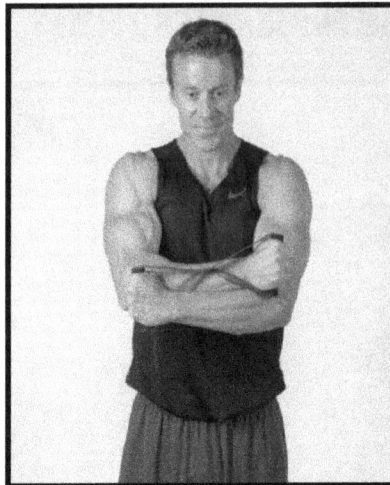

PHASE TWO MON, WED, FRI.

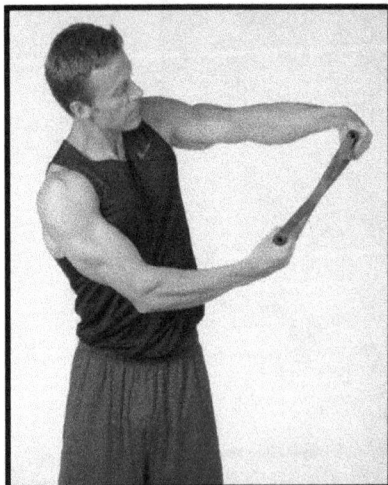

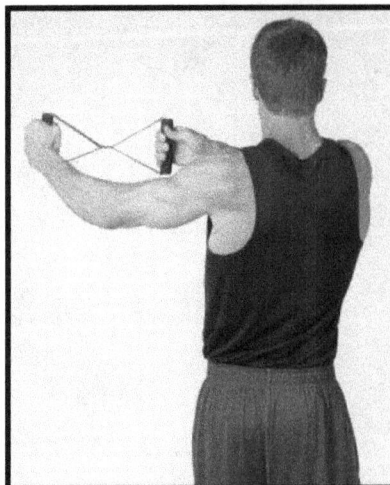

PHASE TWO

11 PHASE TWO

TUESDAY, THURSDAY, SATURDAY

Perform a 20 second Isometric contraction, 3 sets each before moving to the next exercise. Perform each exercise using 50% of force.

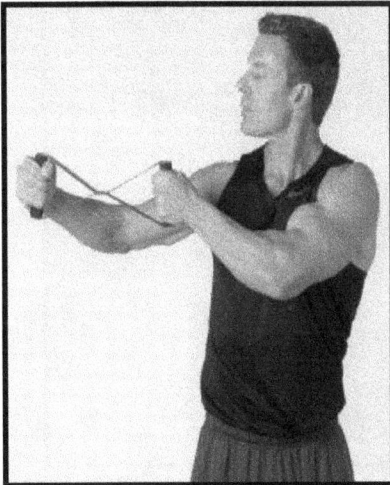
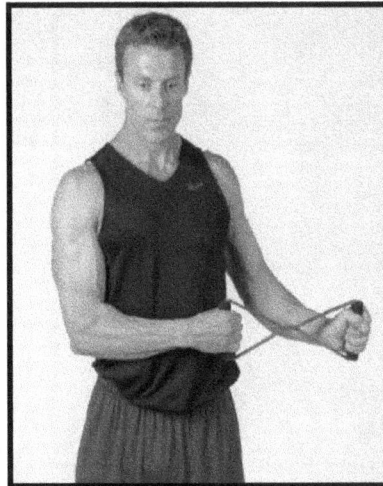
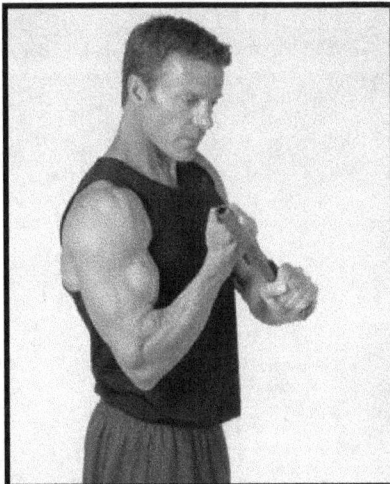
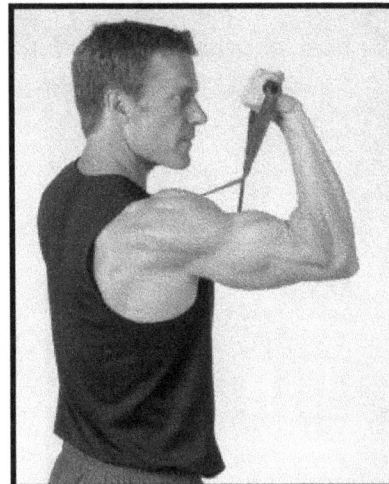

PHASE TWO

11 PHASE TWO

TUESDAY, THURSDAY, SATURDAY

ROUTINE CONTINUED..........

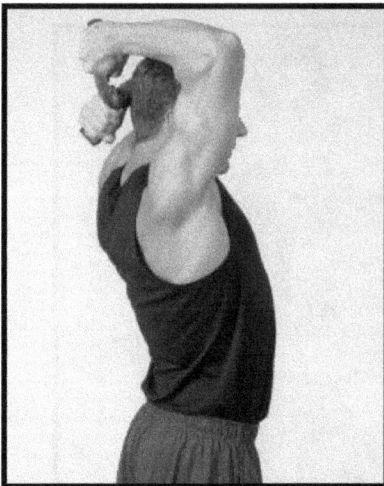
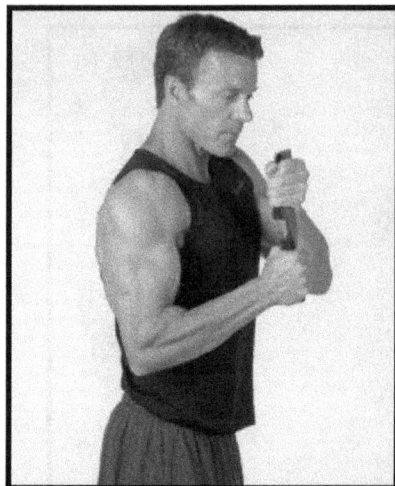

PHASE TWO   TUES, THURS, SAT.

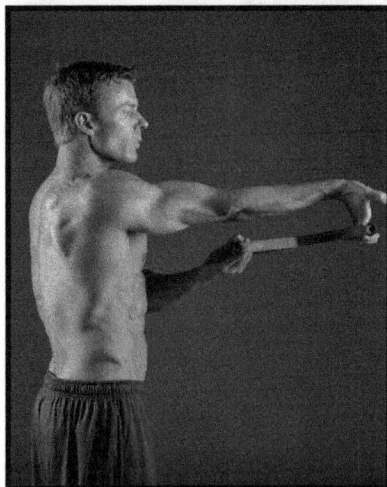
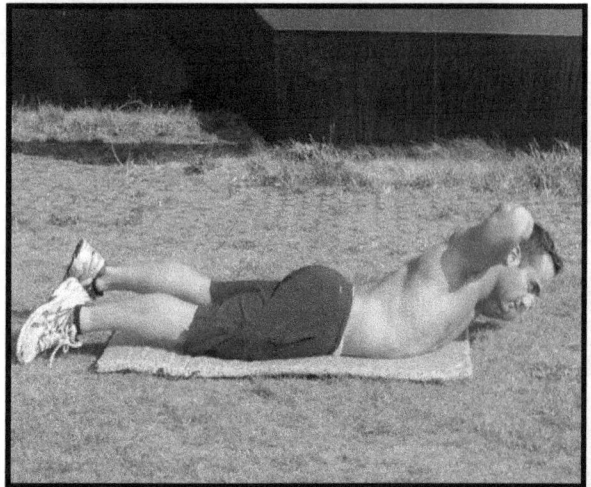

Chapter 12:

MUSCLE BLAST X4 PUMP

MUSCLE BLAST X4 PUMP METHOD
40 SECOND ISOMETRIC CONTRACTION,
2 WEEKS

X4 PUMP

12 X4 PUMP

HOW TO PERFORM THIS ROUTINE:

Perform 40 Isometric Pulses, 1 second mini contraction per exercise.
Perform three sets each exercise using 50-60% of force.

DAY ONE

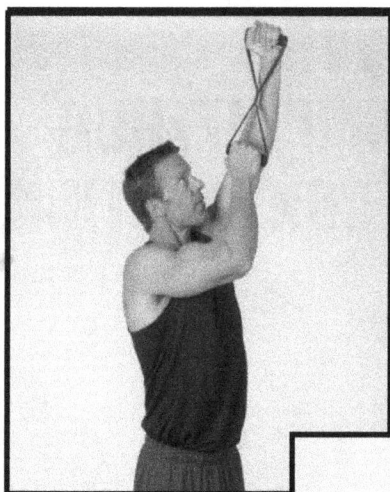
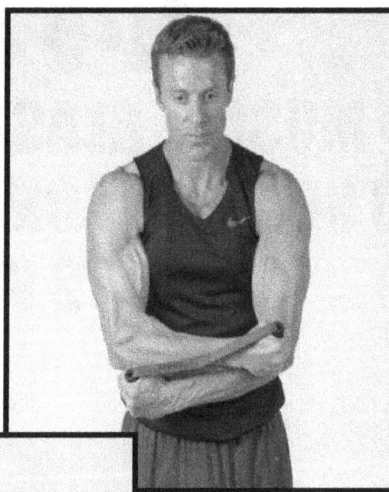
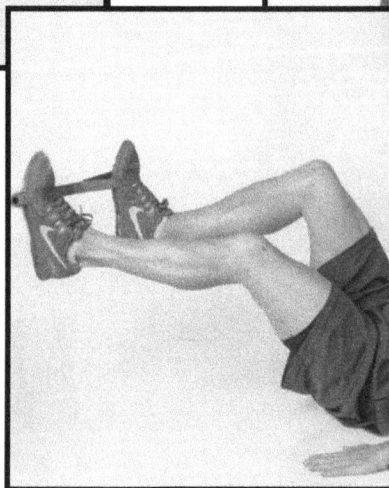

X4 PUMP

12 X4 PUMP

HOW TO PERFORM THIS ROUTINE:

Perform 40 Isometric Pulses, 1 second mini contraction per exercise.
Perform three sets each exercise using 50-60% of force.

DAY ONE continued..........

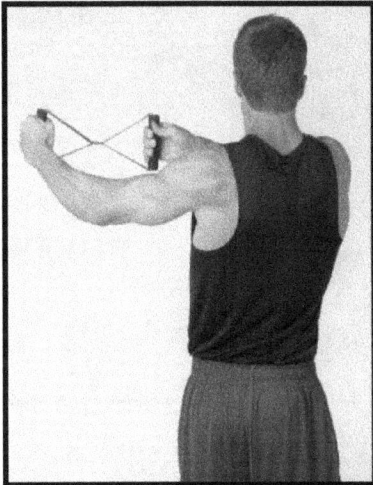

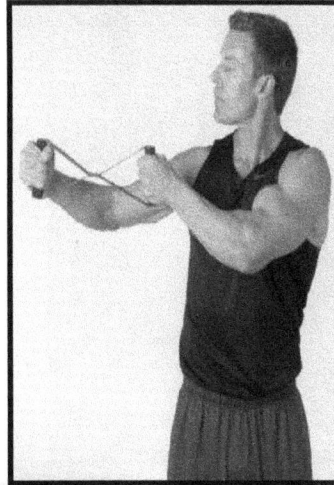

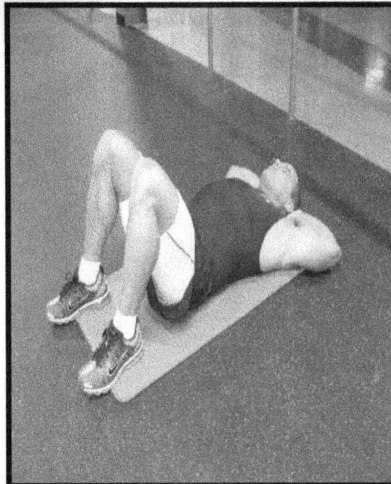

X4 PUMP

12 X4 PUMP

HOW TO PERFORM THIS ROUTINE:
Perform 40 Isometric Pulses, 1 second mini contraction per exercise. Perform three sets each exercise using 50-60% of force.

DAY TWO

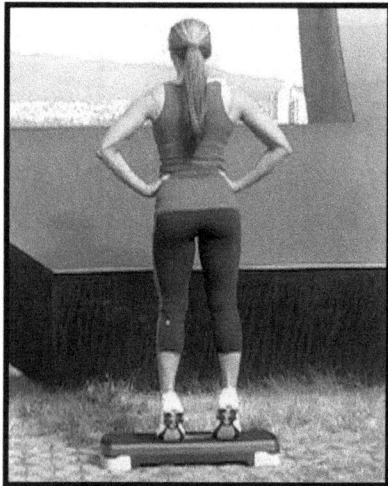

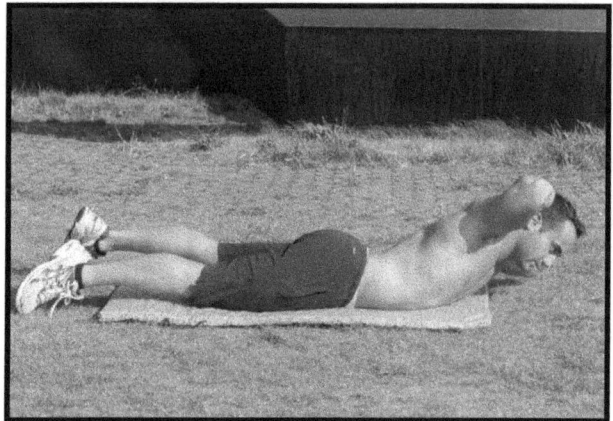

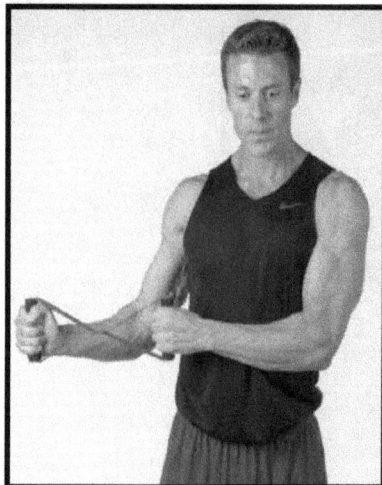

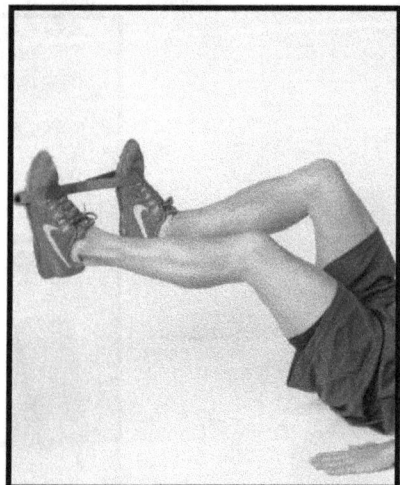

X4 PUMP

12 X4 PUMP

HOW TO PERFORM THIS ROUTINE:

Perform 40 Isometric Pulses, 1 second mini contraction per exercise.
Perform three sets each exercise using 50-60% of force.

DAY TWO continued.............

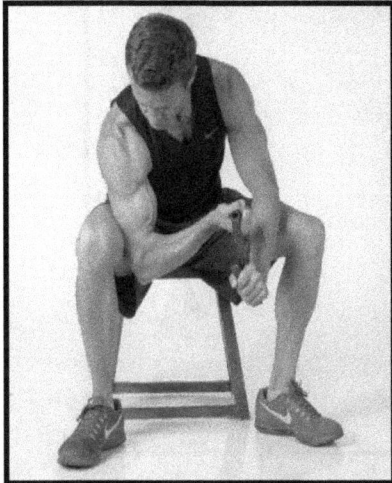

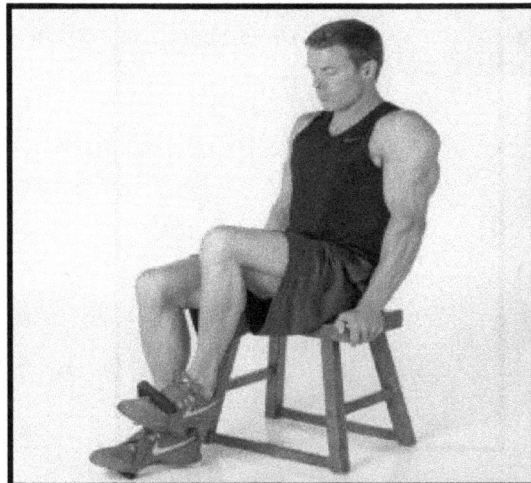

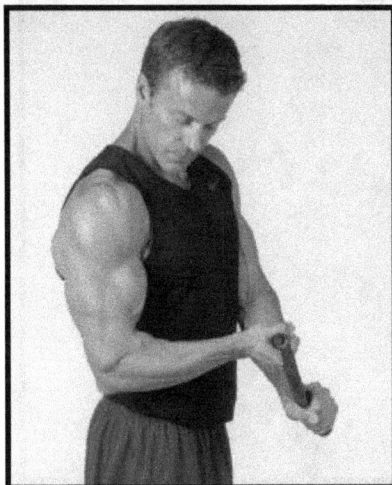

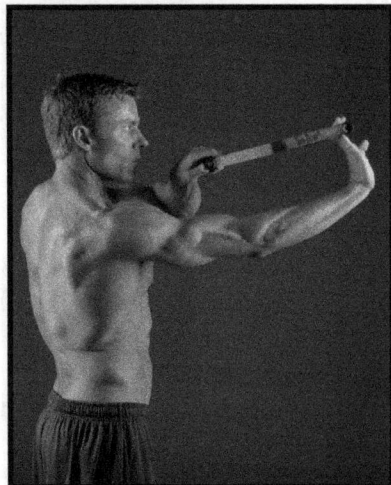

X4 PUMP

12 X4 PUMP

HOW TO PERFORM THIS ROUTINE:

Perform 40 Isometric Pulses, 1 second mini contraction per exercise.
Perform three sets each exercise using 50-60% of force.

DAY THREE

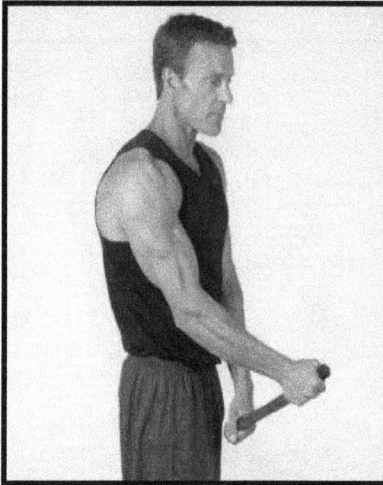
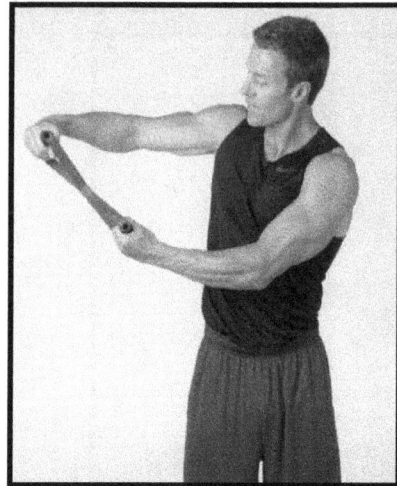

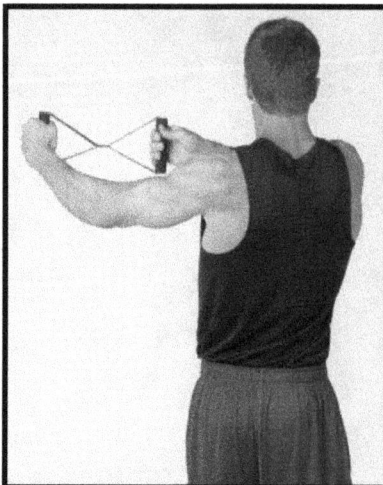
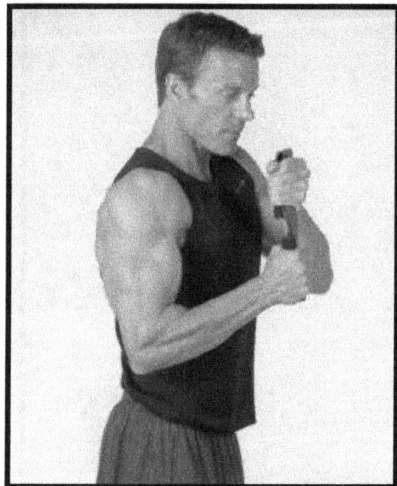

X4 PUMP

12 X4 PUMP

HOW TO PERFORM THIS ROUTINE:

Perform 40 Isometric Pulses, 1 second mini contraction per exercise.
Perform three sets each exercise using 50-60% of force.

DAY THREE continued.......

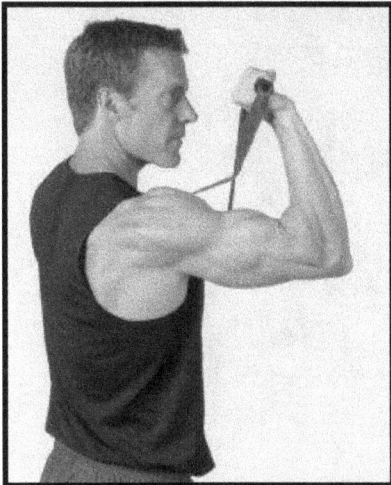

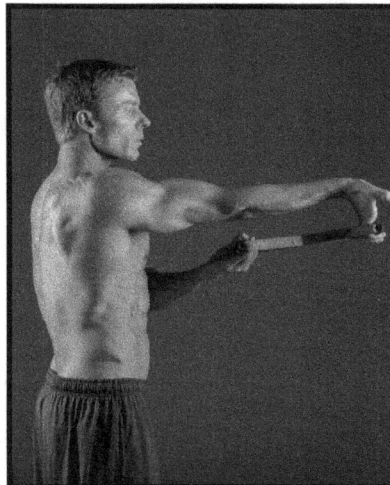

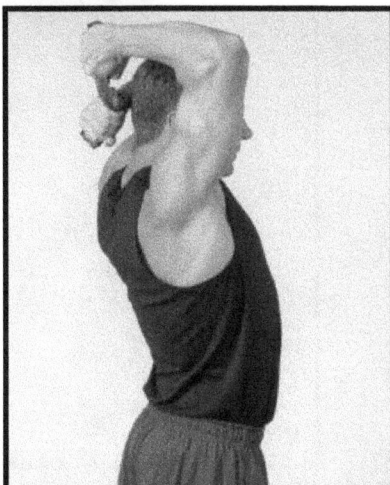

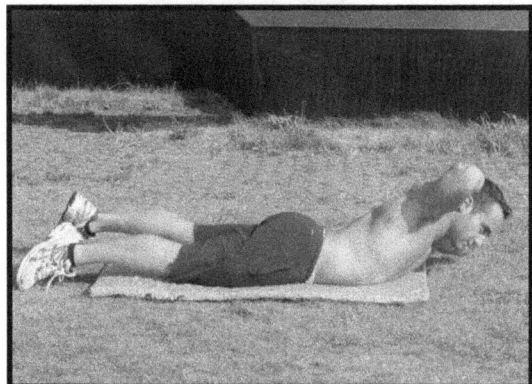

X4 PUMP

12 X4 PUMP

HOW TO PERFORM THIS ROUTINE:
Perform 40 Isometric Pulses, 1 second mini contraction per exercise.
Perform three sets each exercise using 50-60% of force.

DAY THREE continued.......

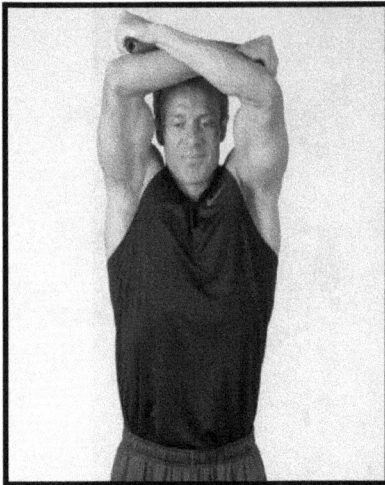

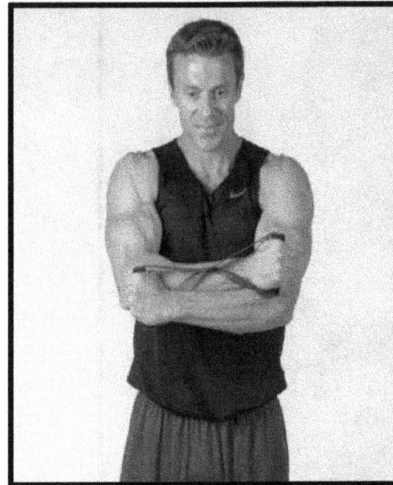

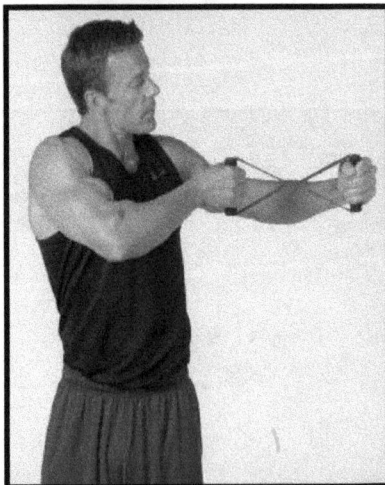

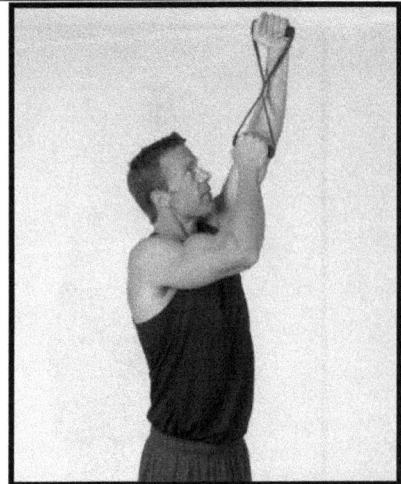

X4 PUMP

12 X4 PUMP

HOW TO PERFORM THIS ROUTINE:

Perform 40 Isometric Pulses, 1 second mini contraction per exercise.
Perform three sets each exercise using 50-60% of force.

DAY FOUR

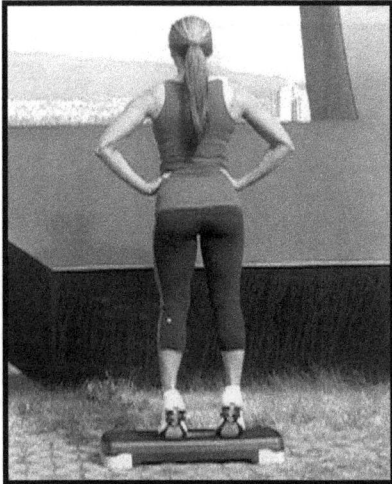

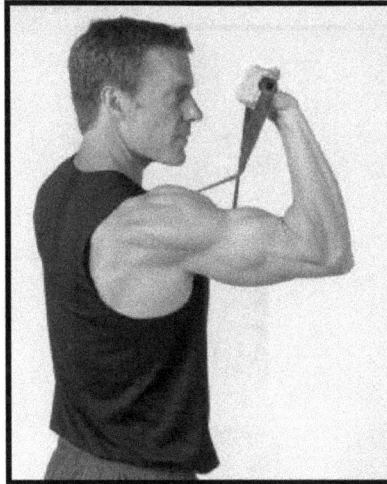

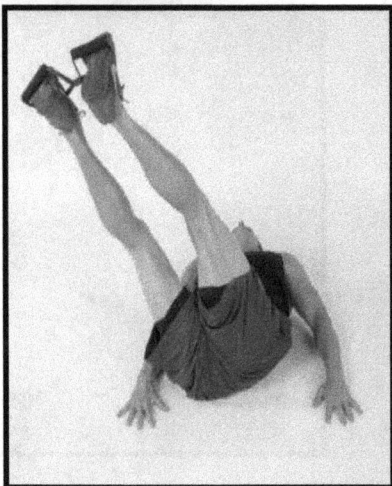

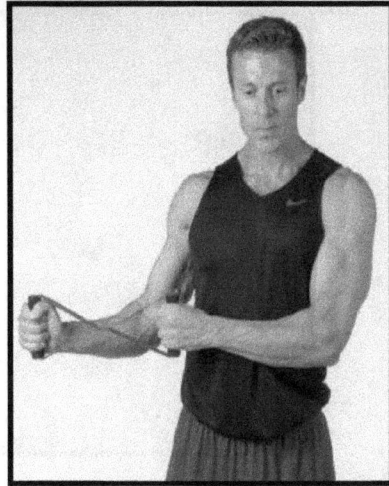

X4 PUMP

12 X4 PUMP

HOW TO PERFORM THIS ROUTINE:

Perform 40 Isometric Pulses, 1 second mini contraction per exercise.
Perform three sets each exercise using 50-60% of force.

DAY FOUR continued......

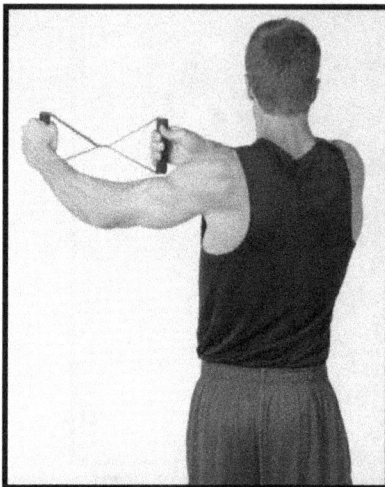

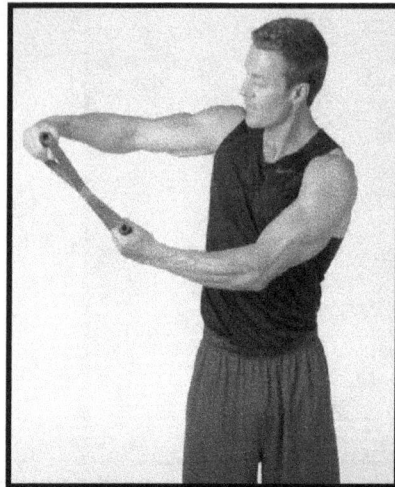

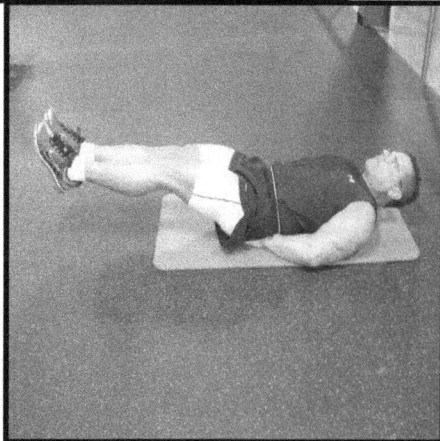

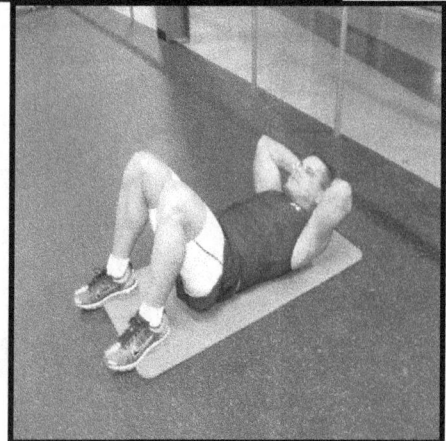

X4 PUMP

12 X4 PUMP

HOW TO PERFORM THIS ROUTINE:

Perform 40 Isometric Pulses, 1 second mini contraction per exercise.
Perform three sets each exercise using 50-60% of force.

DAY FIVE

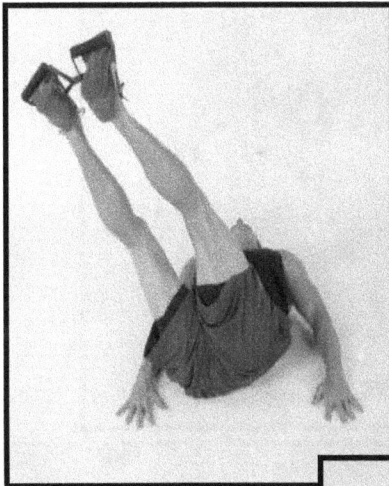

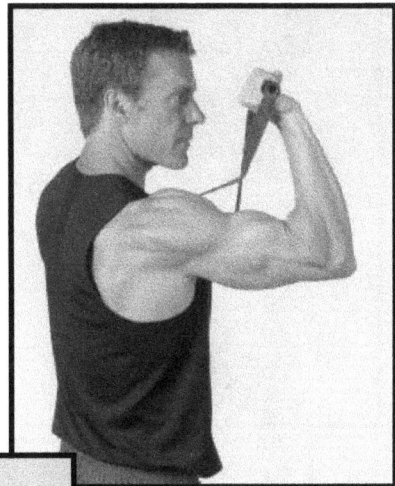

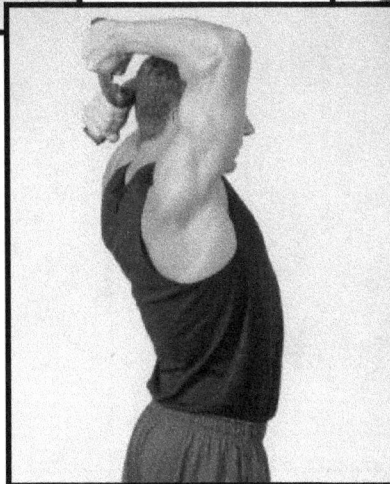

X4 PUMP

12 X4 PUMP

HOW TO PERFORM THIS ROUTINE:

Perform 40 Isometric Pulses, 1 second mini contraction per exercise.
Perform three sets each exercise using 50-60% of force.

DAY FIVE continued.....

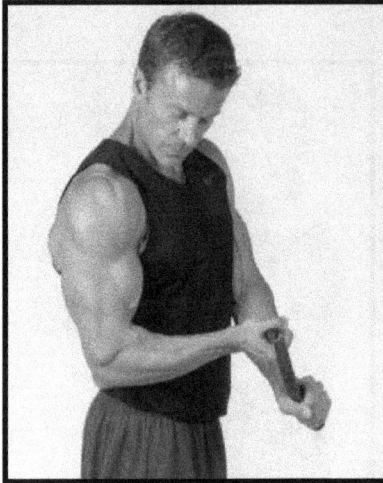
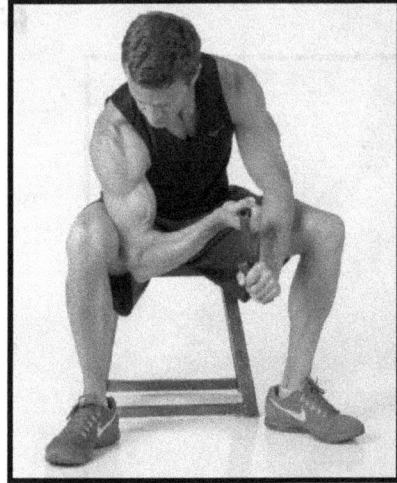
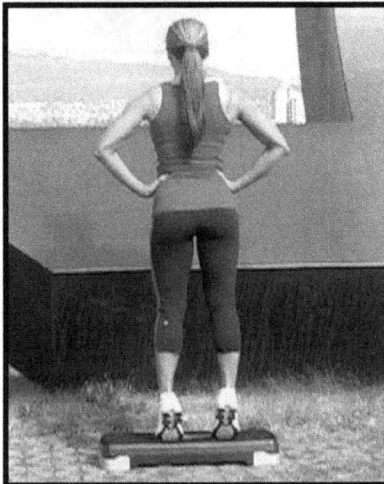
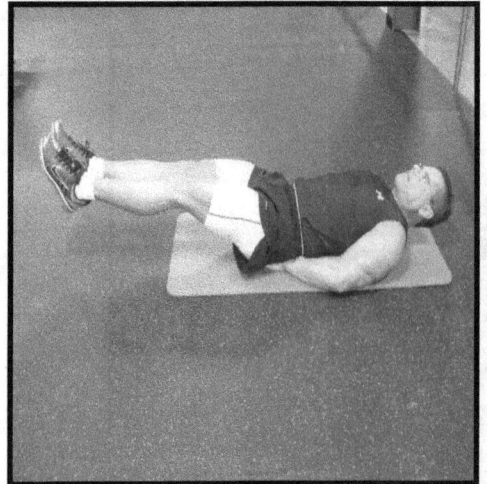

Chapter 13:

THE
MAX FORCE
RIPPED 90
PROGRAM
PHASE ONE

RIPPED 90 PHASE ONE

13 PHASE ONE

HOW TO PERFORM THIS ROUTINE:
RIPPED 90 PHASE ONE

Perform 50 Isometric Pulses, mini contractions at the contracted position. 2-3 sets per exercise. **PERFORM PROGRAM FOR 2 WEEKS**

DAY ONE

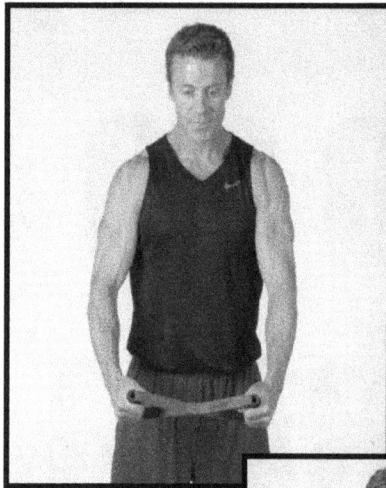
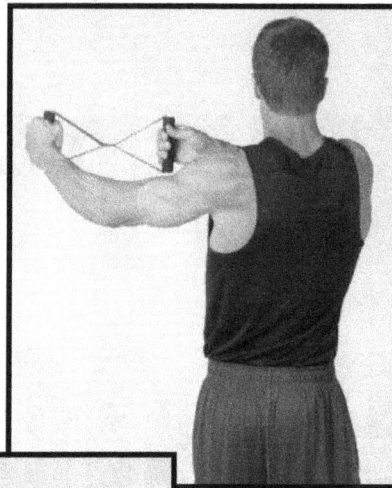
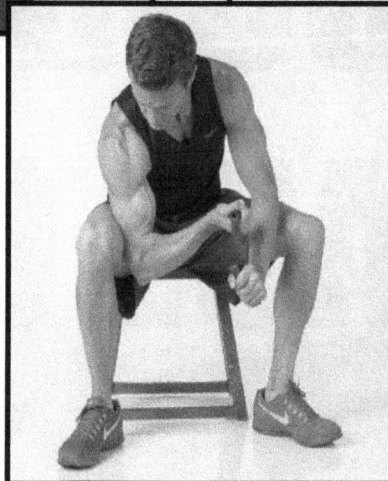

RIPPED 90 PHASE ONE

13 PHASE ONE

HOW TO PERFORM THIS ROUTINE:
RIPPED 90 PHASE ONE

Perform 50 Isometric Pulses, mini contractions at the contracted position. 2-3 sets per exercise. **PERFORM PROGRAM FOR 2 WEEKS**

DAY ONE continued.............

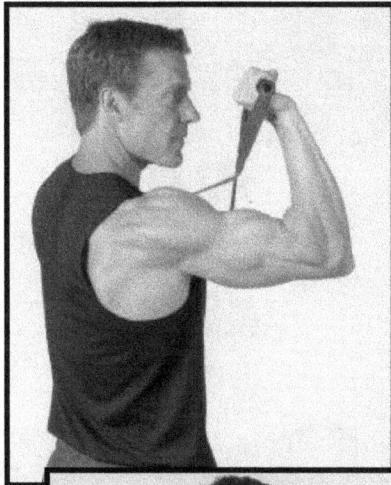

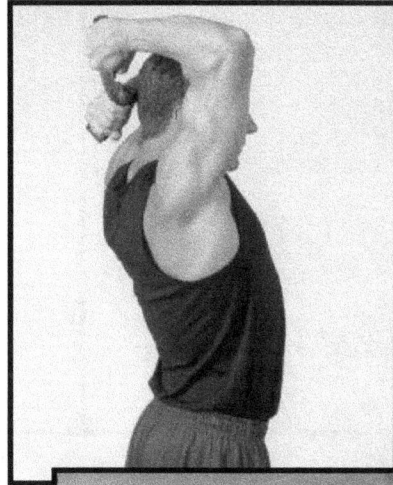

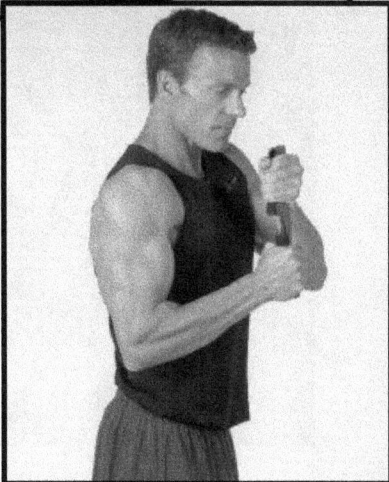

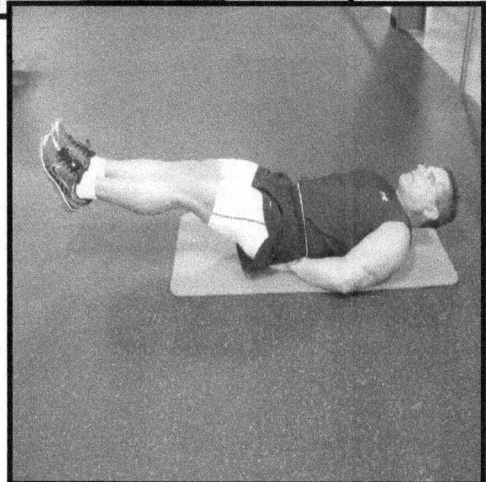

RIPPED 90 PHASE ONE

13 PHASE ONE

HOW TO PERFORM THIS ROUTINE:
RIPPED 90 PHASE ONE

Perform 50 Isometric Pulses, mini contractions at the contracted position. 2-3 sets per exercise. **PERFORM PROGRAM FOR 2 WEEKS**

DAY TWO

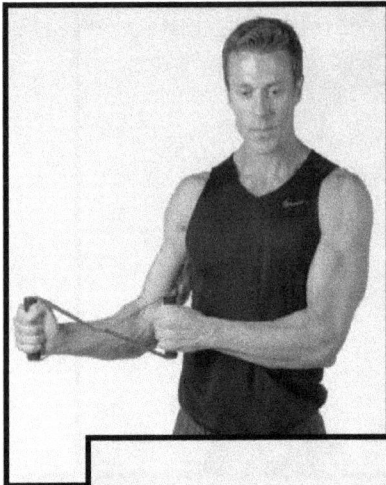

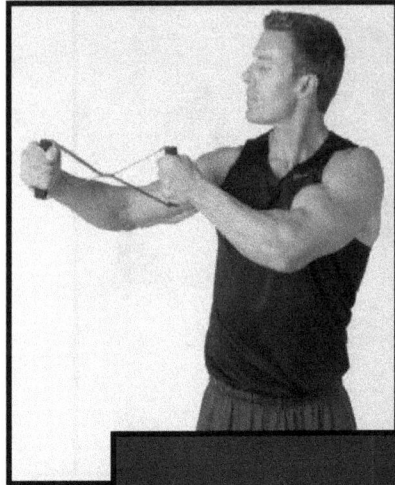

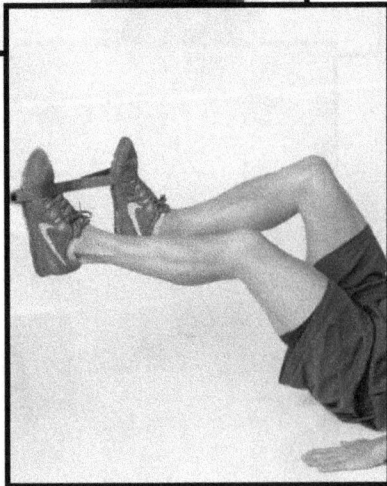

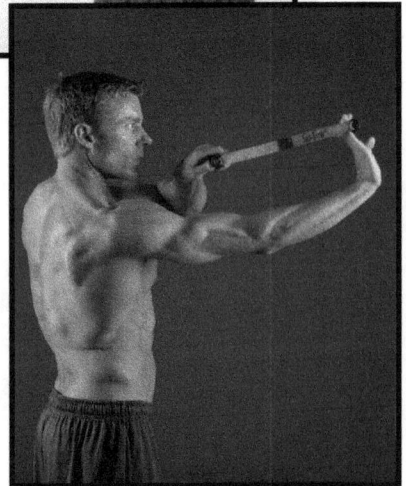

RIPPED 90 PHASE ONE

13 PHASE ONE

HOW TO PERFORM THIS ROUTINE:
RIPPED 90 PHASE ONE

Perform 50 Isometric Pulses, mini contractions at the contracted position. 2-3 sets per exercise. **PERFORM PROGRAM FOR 2 WEEKS**

DAY TWO continued.......

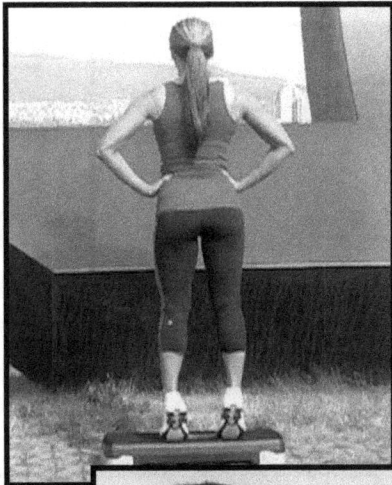
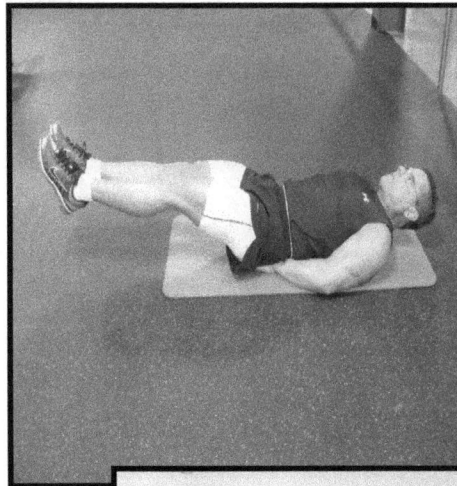
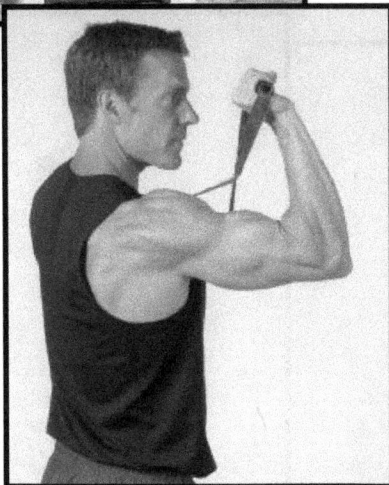
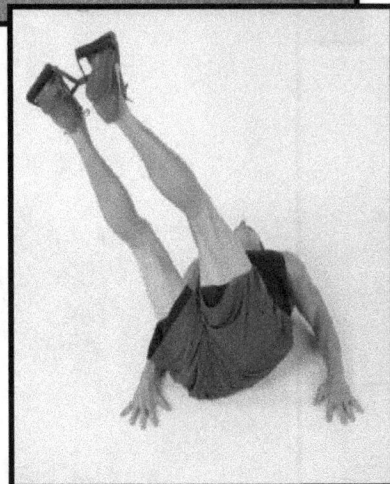

RIPPED 90 PHASE ONE

13 PHASE ONE

HOW TO PERFORM THIS ROUTINE:
RIPPED 90 PHASE ONE

Perform 50 Isometric Pulses, mini contractions at the contracted position. 2-3 sets per exercise. **PERFORM PROGRAM FOR 2 WEEKS**

DAY THREE

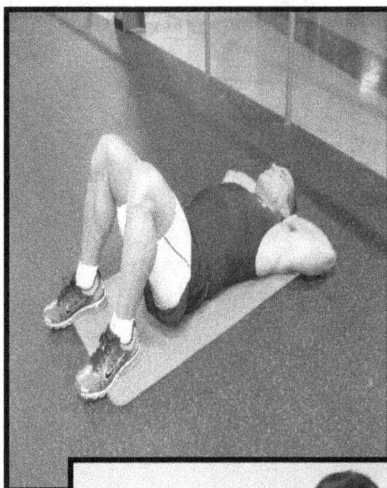
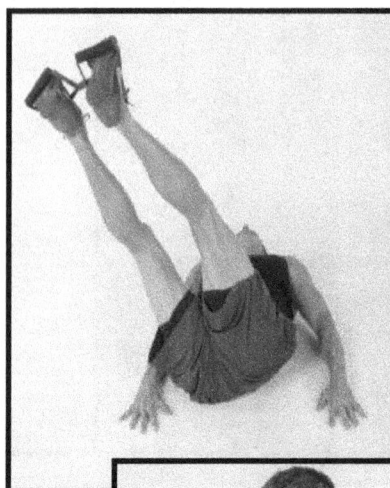
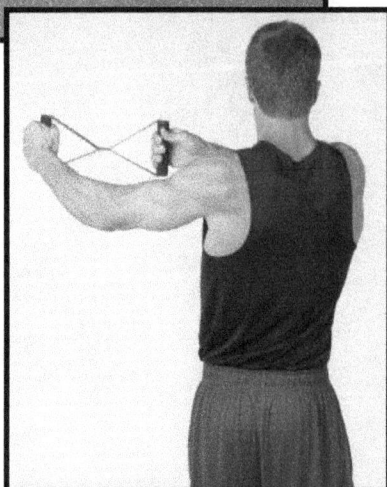
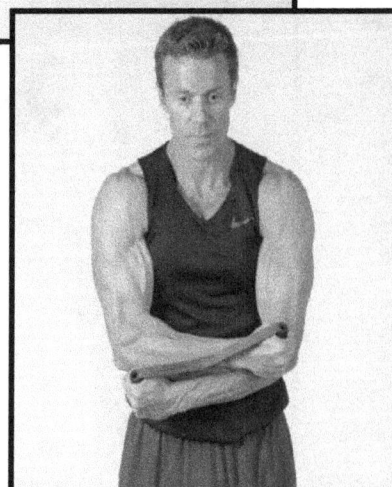

RIPPED 90 PHASE ONE

13 PHASE ONE

HOW TO PERFORM THIS ROUTINE:
RIPPED 90 PHASE ONE

Perform 50 Isometric Pulses, mini contractions at the contracted position. 2-3 sets per exercise. **PERFORM PROGRAM FOR 2 WEEKS**

DAY THREE continued..........

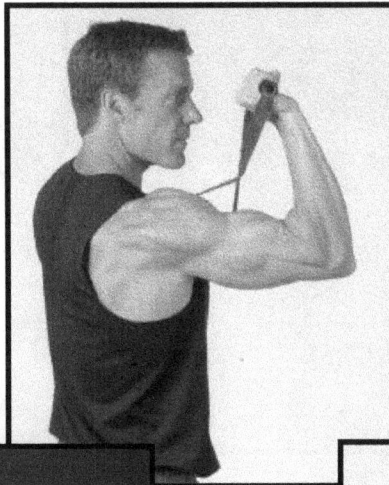

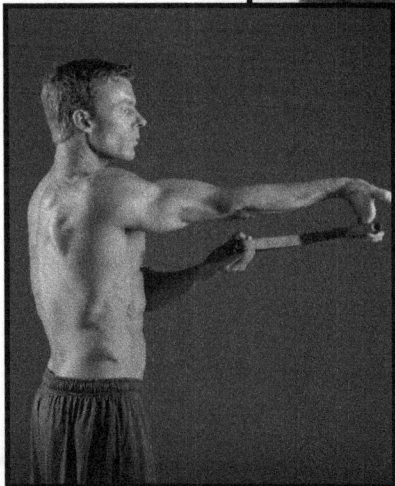

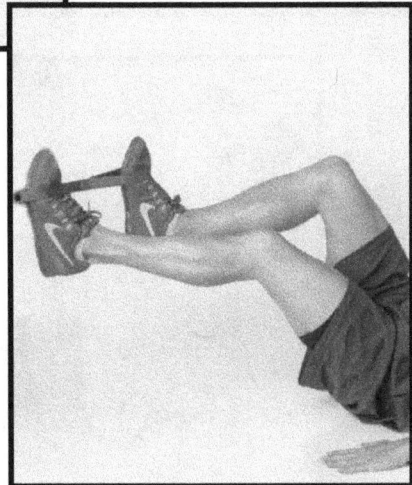

RIPPED 90 PHASE ONE

13 PHASE ONE

HOW TO PERFORM THIS ROUTINE:
RIPPED 90 PHASE ONE

Perform 50 Isometric Pulses, mini contractions at the contracted position. 2-3 sets per exercise. **PERFORM PROGRAM FOR 2 WEEKS**

DAY FOUR

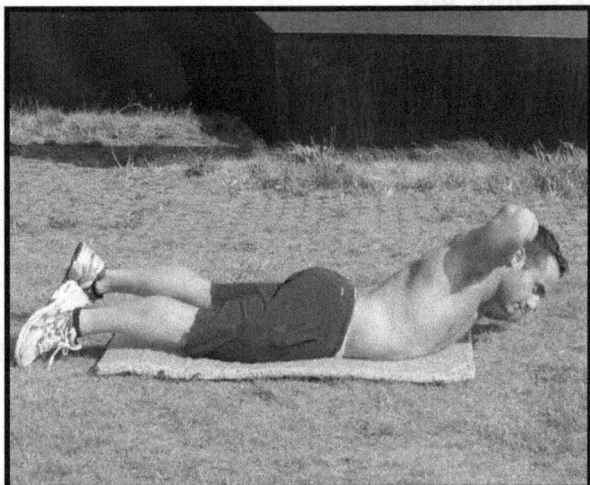

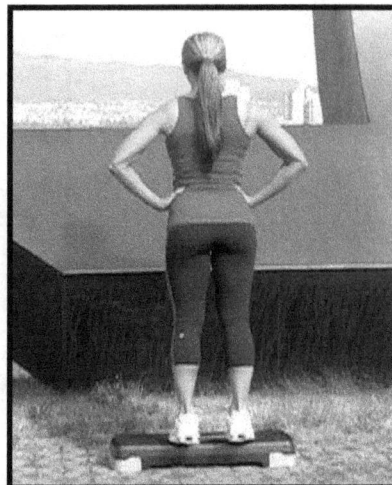

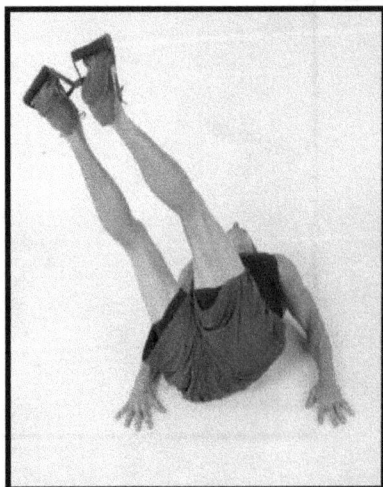

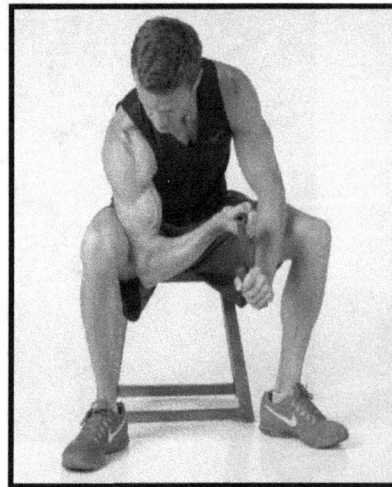

RIPPED 90 PHASE ONE

13 PHASE ONE

HOW TO PERFORM THIS ROUTINE:
RIPPED 90 PHASE ONE

Perform 50 Isometric Pulses, mini contractions at the contracted position. 2-3 sets per exercise. **PERFORM PROGRAM FOR 2 WEEKS**

DAY FIVE

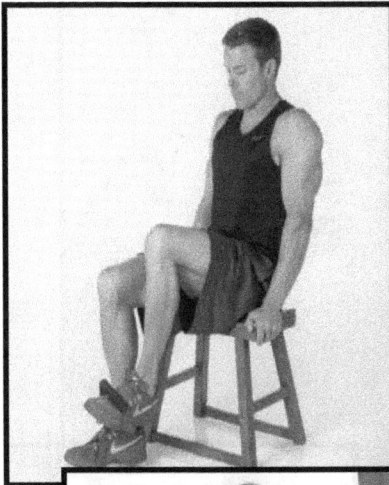
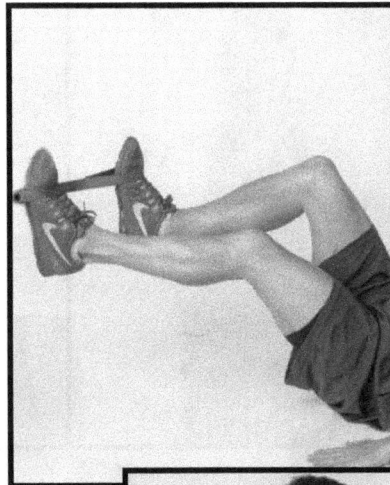
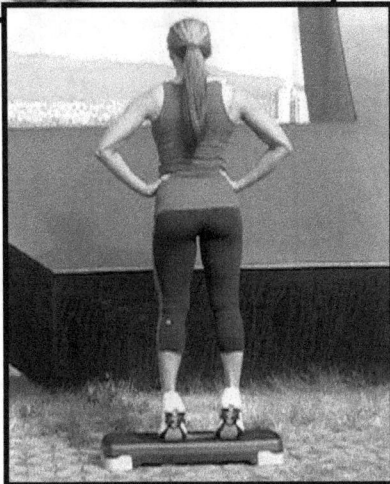
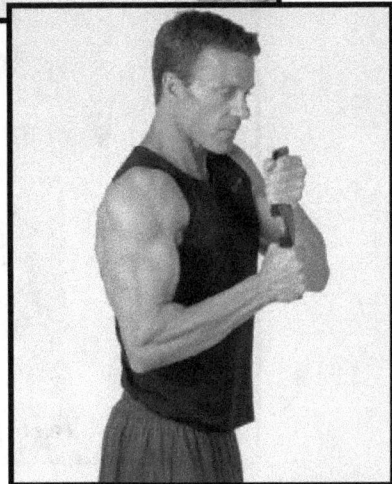

RIPPED 90 PHASE ONE

13 PHASE ONE

HOW TO PERFORM THIS ROUTINE:
RIPPED 90 PHASE ONE

Perform 50 Isometric Pulses, mini contractions at the contracted position.
2-3 sets per exercise. **PERFORM PROGRAM FOR 2 WEEKS**

DAY FIVE continued............

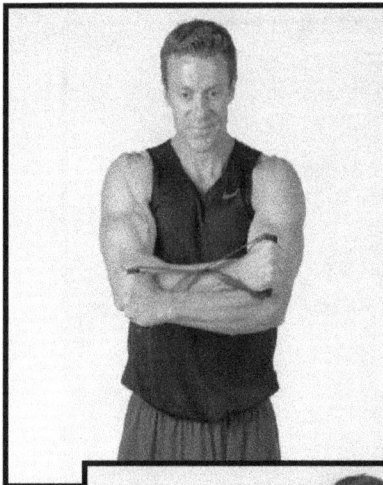

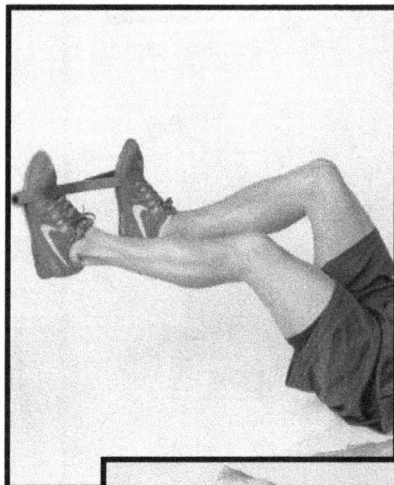

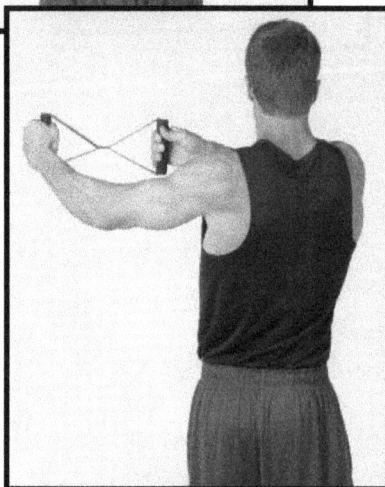

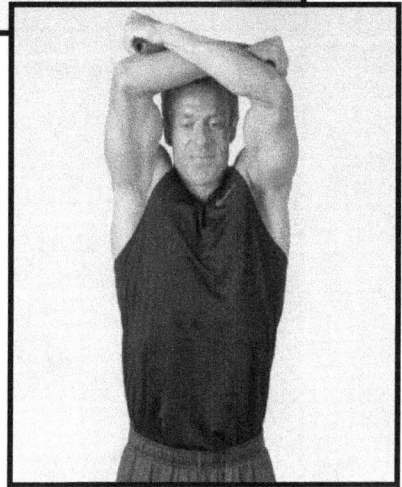

Chapter 13:

THE MAX FORCE RIPPED 90 PROGRAM PHASE TWO

PHASE TWO

13 RIPPED 90

HOW TO PERFORM THIS ROUTINE:
PHASE TWO

Perform an isometric hold for 30 seconds. Alternate day one and day two for 6 days per week. Five sets per exercise. Perform this program for 3 weeks, rest time 5 seconds between sets. **PERFORM PROGRAM FOR 2 WEEKS**

DAY ONE

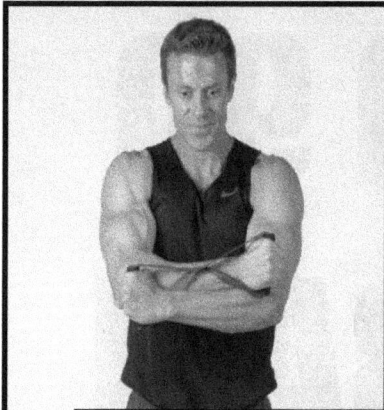

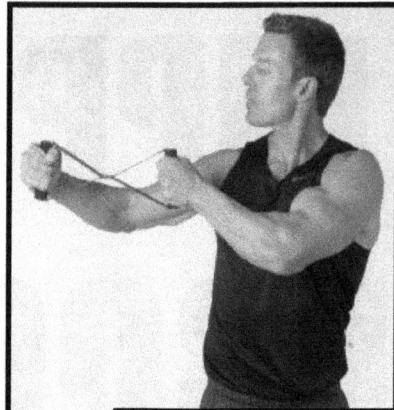

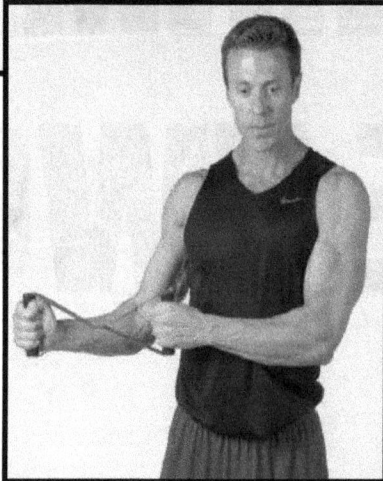

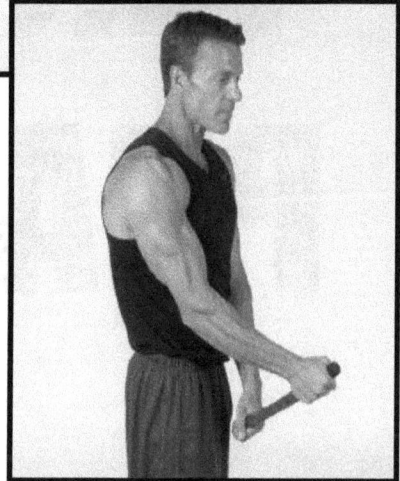

PHASE TWO

13 RIPPED 90

HOW TO PERFORM THIS ROUTINE:
PHASE TWO

Perform an isometric hold for 30 seconds. Alternate day one and day two 6 days per week. One set per exercise. Perform this program for 2 weeks.

DAY ONE continued..........

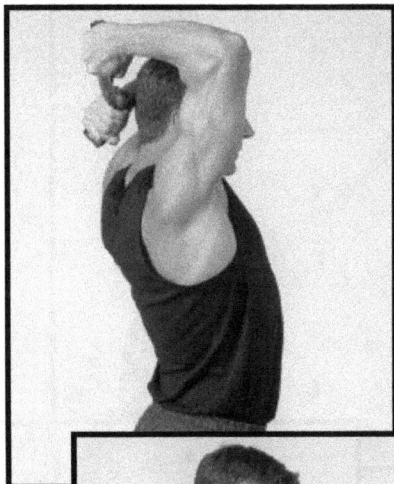

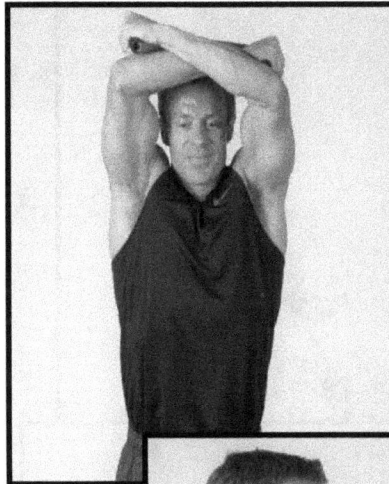

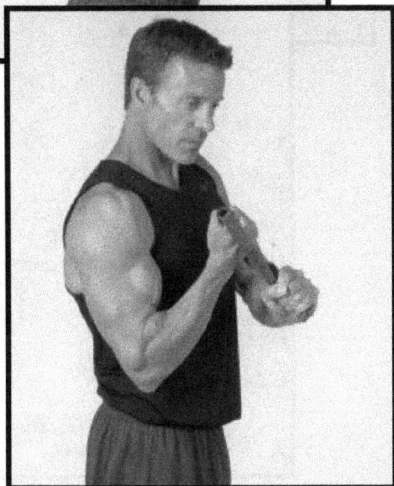

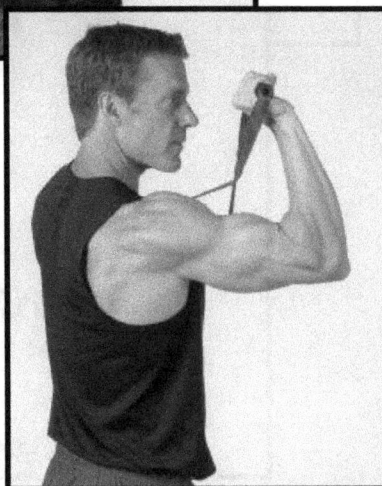

PHASE TWO

13 RIPPED 90

HOW TO PERFORM THIS ROUTINE:
PHASE TWO

Perform an isometric hold for 30 seconds. Alternate day one and day two 6 days per week. One set per exercise. Perform this program for 2 weeks.

DAY TWO

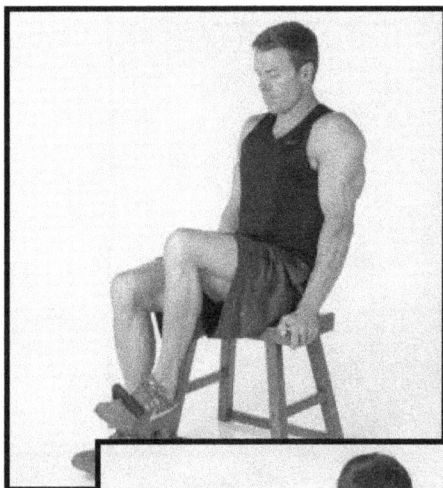
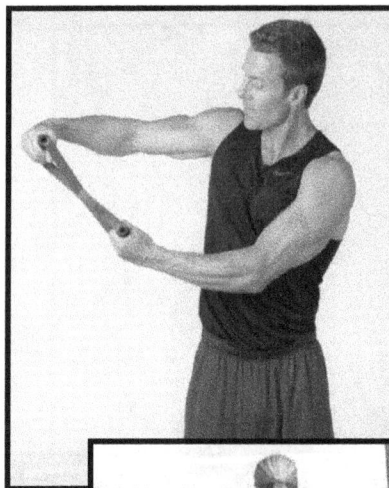
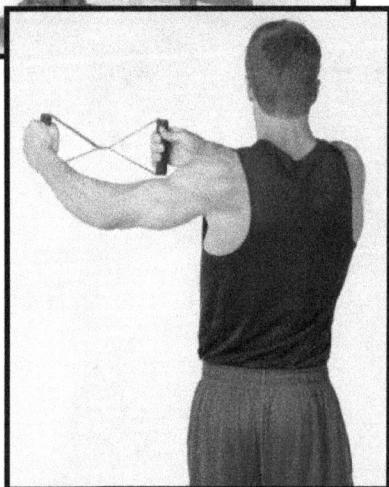
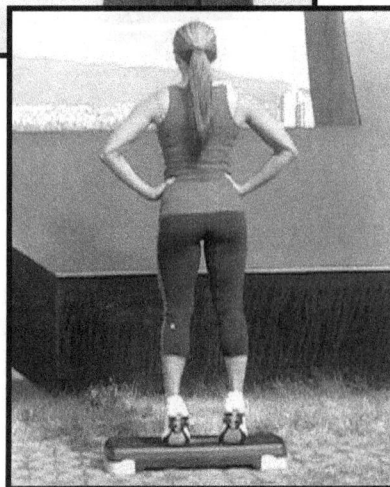

PHASE TWO

13 RIPPED 90

HOW TO PERFORM THIS ROUTINE:
PHASE TWO

Perform an isometric hold for 30 seconds. Alternate day one and day two 6 days per week. One set per exercise. Perform this program for 2 weeks.

DAY TWO continued........

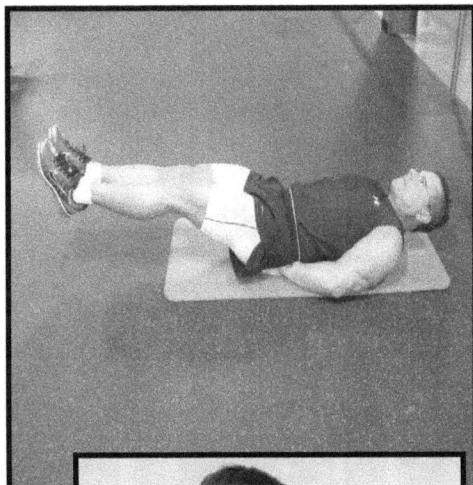
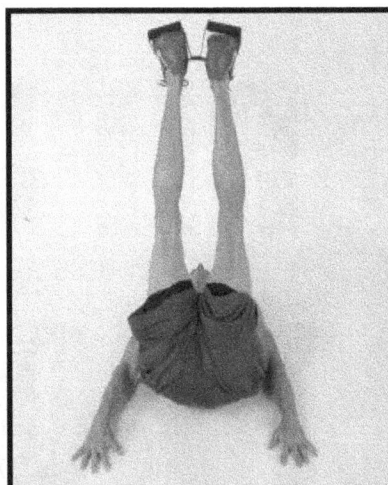
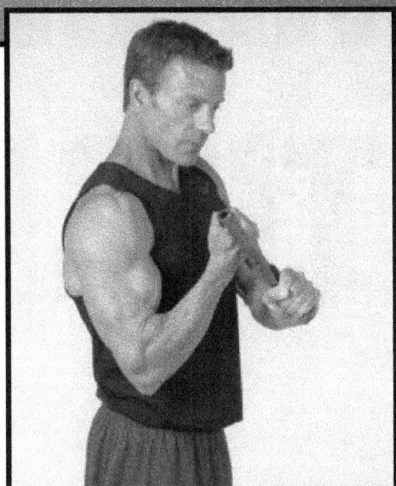
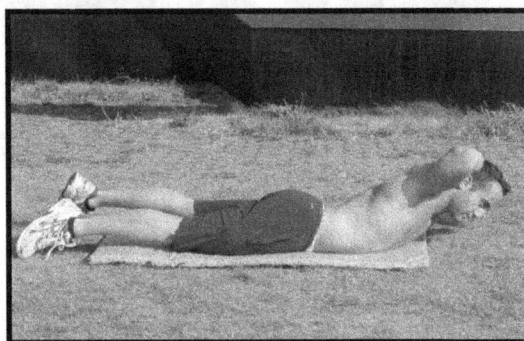

Chapter 13:

THE
MAX FORCE
RIPPED 90
PROGRAM
PHASE THREE

PHASE THREE

13 RIPPED 90

HOW TO PERFORM THIS ROUTINE:
PHASE THREE

Perform 20 Isometric Pulses, 4 sets each exercise. Alternate day one and day two for 6 days per week. **PERFORM PROGRAM FOR 2 WEEKS**

DAY ONE

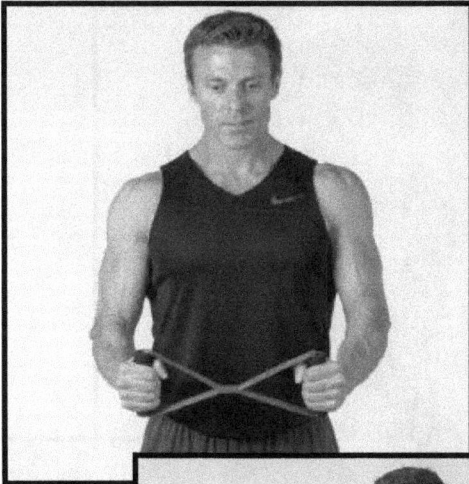
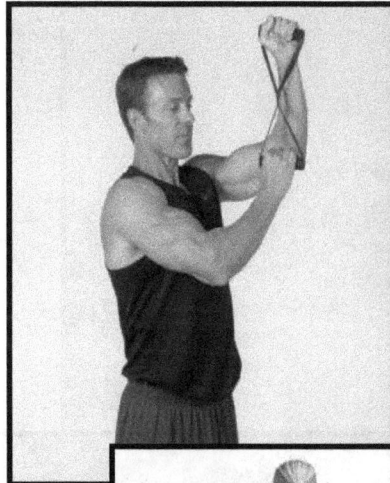
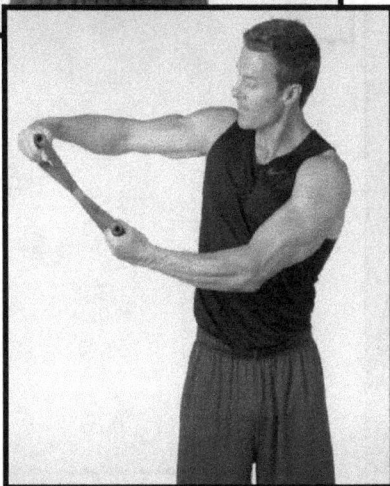
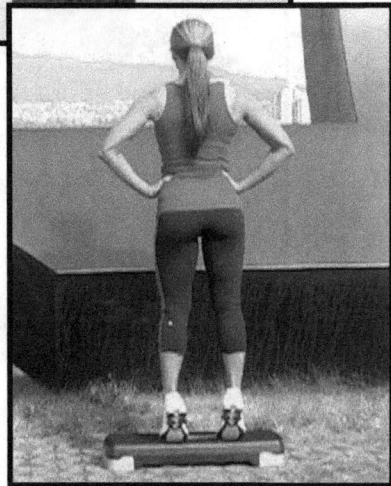

PHASE THREE

13 RIPPED 90

HOW TO PERFORM THIS ROUTINE:
PHASE THREE

Perform a 20 second isometric contraction, 4 sets each exercise. Alternate day one and day two for 6 days per week.

DAY ONE continued...........

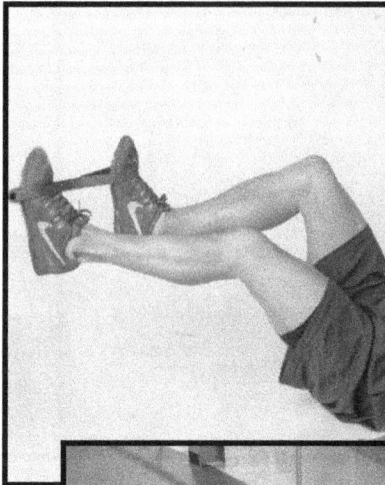

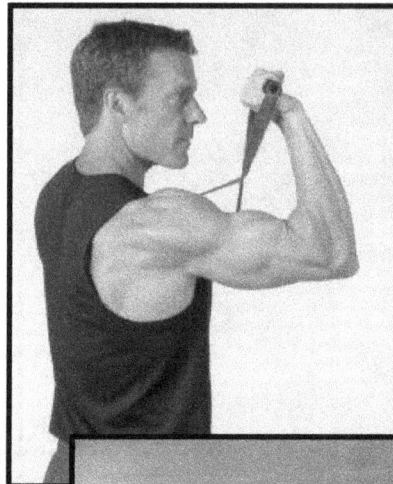

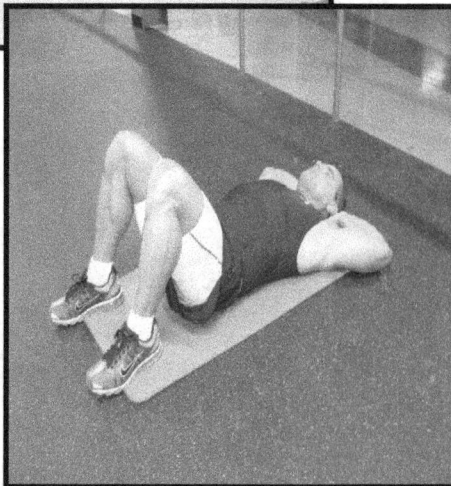

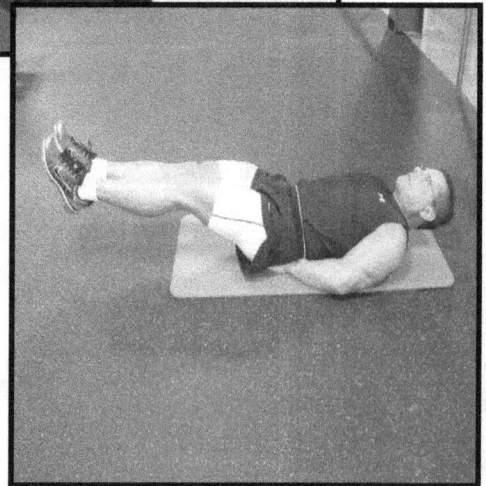

PHASE THREE

13 RIPPED 90

HOW TO PERFORM THIS ROUTINE:
PHASE THREE

Perform a 20 second isometric contraction, 4 sets each exercise. Alternate day one and day two for 6 days per week.

DAY TWO

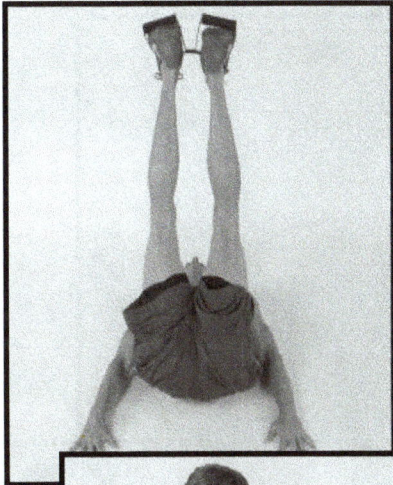

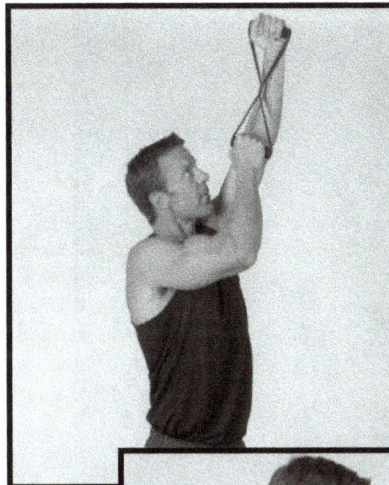

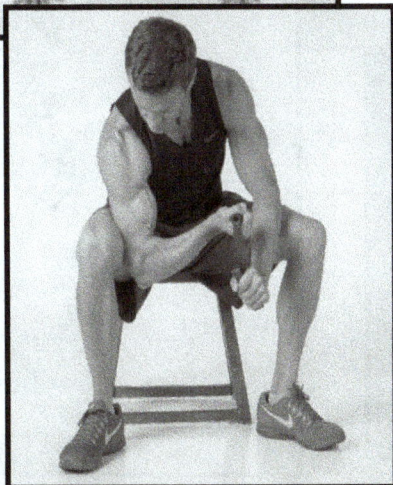

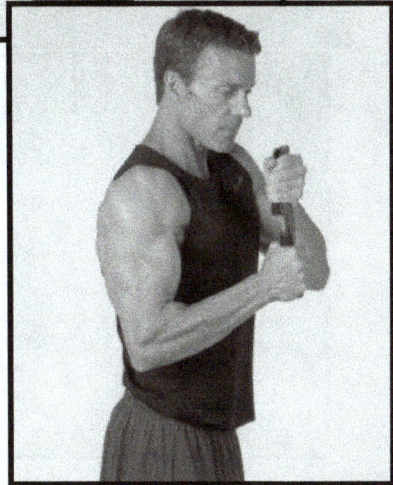

PHASE THREE

13 RIPPED 90

HOW TO PERFORM THIS ROUTINE:
PHASE THREE

Perform a 20 second isometric contraction, 4 sets each exercise. Alternate day one and day two for 6 days per week.

DAY TWO continued..........

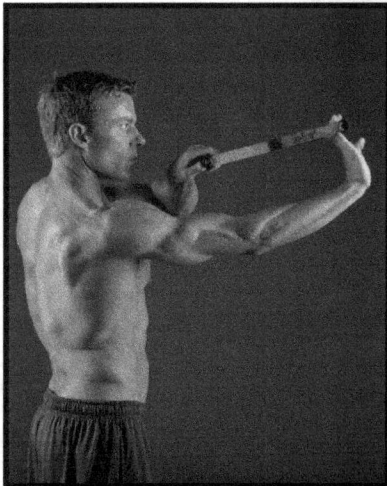

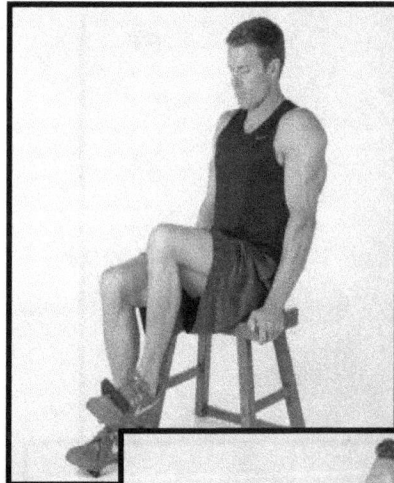

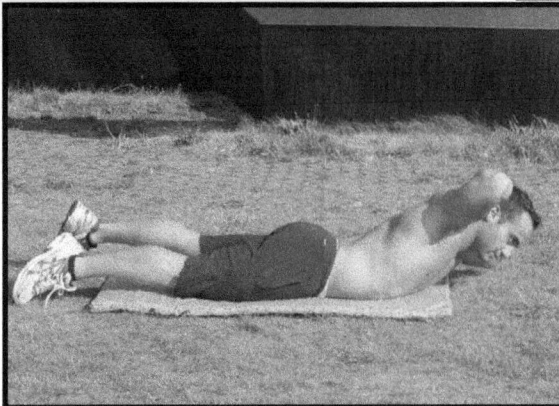

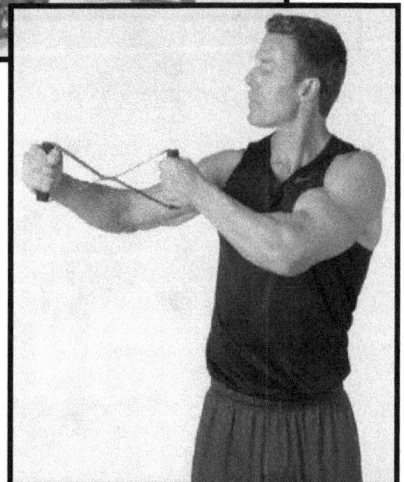

We are looking forward to hearing from you on your progress.
Please drop us an email skippymarl@icloud. com

www.ingramcontent.com/pod-product-compliance
Lightning Source LLC
Chambersburg PA
CBHW081403270326
41930CB00015B/3397

9 781990 089053